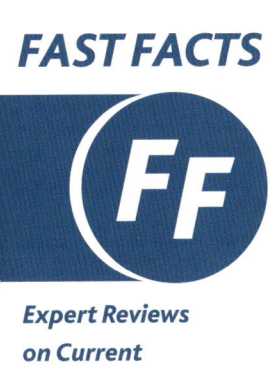

FAST FACTS

Expert Reviews on Current Research

Rheumatology Highlights 2003–04

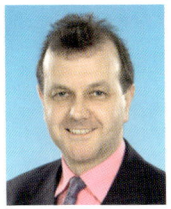

Edited by John D Isaacs PhD FRCP
Professor of Clinical Rheumatology,
University of Newcastle upon Tyne, UK

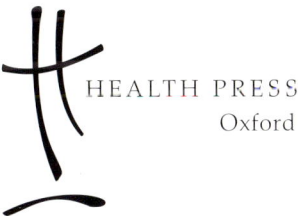

Fast Facts – Rheumatology Highlights 2003–04
First published April 2004

© 2004 Health Press Limited
Health Press Limited, Elizabeth House, Queen Street, Abingdon,
Oxford OX14 3JR, UK
Tel: +44 (0)1235 523233
Fax: +44 (0)1235 523238

Book orders can be placed by telephone or via the website.
For regional distributors or to order via the website, please go to:
www.fastfacts.com
For telephone orders, please call 01752 202301 (UK) or
800 538 1287 (North America, toll free).

Fast Facts is a trademark of Health Press Limited.

All rights reserved. No part of this publication may be reproduced, stored in a retrieval system, or transmitted in any form or by any means, electronic, mechanical, photocopying, recording or otherwise, without the express permission of the publisher.

The publisher and the authors have made every effort to ensure the accuracy of this book, but cannot accept responsibility for any errors or omissions.

Registered names, trademarks, etc. used in this book, even when not marked as such, are not to be considered unprotected by law.

A CIP catalogue record for this title is available from the British Library.

ISBN 1-90373449-5

Isaacs, JD (John)
Fast Facts – Rheumatology Highlights 2003–04/
John D Isaacs

Medical illustrations by Dee McLean, London, UK.
Typesetting and page layout by Zed, Oxford, UK.
Printed by Fine Print (Services) Ltd, Oxford, UK.
Cover image reproduced courtesy of Dr G Hide,
University of Newcastle upon Tyne, UK

Printed with vegetable inks on fully biodegradable and recyclable paper manufactured from sustainable forests.

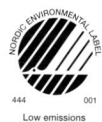
Low emissions during production

Low chlorine

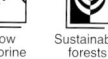
Sustainable forests

Introduction	5
Osteoarthritis *Marc C Hochberg MD MPH*	7
Osteoporosis and bone *Steven R Goldring MD*	15
Systemic lupus erythematosus *Bevra H Hahn MD*	25
Scleroderma *Christopher P Denton PhD FRCP*	32
Vasculitis treatment *David Jayne MD FRCP*	44
The spondyloarthritides *Juergen Braun MD and Joachim Sieper MD*	52
Psoriatic arthritis *Adrian N Gibbs MB MRCPI and Douglas J Veale MD FRCPI FRCP*	63
Juvenile idiopathic arthritis *Kiran Nistala BA MSc MRCP and Tauny Southwood BM BS FRACP FRCPA FRCP FRCPCH*	70
Cytokine blockade *Henry Townsend MD and Larry Moreland MD*	81
Targeting lymphocytes using biological therapies *John D Isaacs PhD FRCP*	89
From genetics to functional genomics *Anna Lucia Bernardini MD and Salvatore Albani MD PhD*	97
Mesenchymal progenitor cells *Elena Jones PhD, Anne English FIBMS and Dennis McGonagle PhD FRCPI*	105

Introduction

The 1990s will be remembered in rheumatology circles for the clinical application of tumor necrosis factor α blockade in rheumatoid arthritis (RA). The start of the 21st century promises to be just as exciting, however, as highlighted in this volume. Other cytokine targets are emerging in RA (see Townsend and Moreland) but, crucially, potentially pivotal cytokines are also being identified in other diseases. These include interferon β in systemic lupus erythematosus (SLE) and transforming growth factor β in scleroderma (see Hahn and Denton, respectively). Furthermore, tolerogenic therapies, which could actually switch off autoreactivity, are currently in clinical trial in SLE and RA (see Hahn and Isaacs, respectively). Meanwhile, conventional treatment algorithms are being challenged in SLE (see Hahn) and vasculitis (see Jayne), and progress in disease classification and assessment is improving the sensitivity of clinical trials, with imaging playing an increasingly important role (see Denton; Nistala and Southwood; Gibbs and Veale; Braun and Sieper; and Hochberg).

New treatment paradigms arise from novel pathogenetic insights. Recent examples include endothelin receptor blockade in scleroderma and the use of parathyroid hormone to treat osteoporosis (see Denton and Goldring, respectively). Similarly, the realization that osteoarthritis is not simply 'wear and tear' means that disease modification is now a viable therapeutic goal in that condition (see Hochberg). Recent genetic discoveries underline the importance of immunoregulation in autoimmunity, and have suggested novel pathogenetic pathways in RA (see Bernardini and Albani). Finally, tissue repair by mesenchymal progenitor cells may facilitate the regeneration of damaged joints and provide the next quantum leap in rheumatic disease therapeutics (see Jones, English and McGonagle).

John Isaacs
Editor

Osteoarthritis

Marc C Hochberg MD MPH
University of Maryland School of Medicine, Baltimore, USA

Osteoarthritis (OA) is the most common form of arthritis. OA, when it involves the hip and/or knee, accounts for more functional limitation and physical disability than any other chronic disease among adults, and is the most common indication for total hip and total knee replacement. It is estimated that the costs associated with OA exceed 2% of the gross national product in developed countries.

Risk factors for the development and/or progression of OA have been identified in epidemiological studies and can be broadly divided into systemic factors that increase the susceptibility to OA and local biomechanical factors that influence the development of OA at a particular joint (Table 1).[1]

Pathogenesis
OA is now recognized to be a disorder that affects all the tissues of the diarthrodial joint, including the articular cartilage, subchondral bone, synovium and periarticular soft tissues. While the pathology of OA has long been characterized by degradation of the articular cartilage, recent work has identified the important role of the chondrocyte in the synthesis of both the matrix components and the enzymes that degrade the matrix.[2] Chondrocytes can be activated by mechanical stimulation and inflammatory cytokines, particularly interleukin (IL)-1, to produce degradative enzymes as well as cytokines and small proinflammatory molecules, including nitric oxide and prostaglandins. In addition, chondrocytes can respond to growth factors, including insulin-like growth factor-1 and transforming growth factor-β, that act to increase the synthesis of matrix components; these anabolic effects of growth factors, however, can be blunted by IL-1.

TABLE 1

Risk factors for osteoarthritis

Systemic factors	Local factors
• Age	• Obesity
• Sex	• Joint injury
• Ethnicity	• Joint deformity
• Genes	– acquired
• Bone mass/density	– congenital
• Nutritional	• Muscle weakness
• Metabolic	• Joint inflammation
• Others	• Occupation

Attention has been redirected to the subchondral bone as an important component of the disease process; indeed, remodeling of subchondral trabecular bone and calcified cartilage with increased bone turnover and reduced subchondral bone mineral density may contribute to the development of OA.[3] The reduction in this excessive remodeling of the subchondral plate may explain, in part, the apparent beneficial effects of the nitrogen-containing bisphosphonates risedronate and alendronate in preventing the development of OA in the Duncan-Hartley guinea pig and the rat anterior cruciate ligament transection models of OA, respectively. Finally, the role of inflammation in the progression of OA has been reemphasized by the findings of synovitis on arthroscopy and magnetic resonance imaging (MRI), elevations in serum levels of acute-phase reactants (e.g. C-reactive protein), and evidence of activation and expression of cytokine and other proinflammatory genes in synoviocytes and mononuclear cells obtained from synovial biopsies and peripheral blood.[4–6]

Imaging

The role of MRI in the assessment of OA of the knee has increased. This technique is more sensitive than conventional radiography in detecting cartilage lesions and bony changes, and is a highly reliable quantitative measure of cartilage volume both cross-sectionally and longitudinally.[7] Bone-marrow lesions, referred to as 'bone marrow edema', are associated with knee pain and an increased risk of progression of radiographic knee OA as defined by joint-space narrowing.[8,9] Additional findings on MRI that are associated with pain in patients with knee OA include synovial thickening, moderate-to-large effusions and periarticular lesions, including anserine bursitis.[10,11]

Management

The management of patients with OA continues to evolve; treatment options are summarized in Table 2. The treatment approaches to OA were discussed at a conference held at the National Institutes of Health (Bethesda, Maryland, USA) in July 1999.[12] Both the American College of Rheumatology (ACR) and the European League Against Rheumatism (EULAR) published recommendations for the management of OA in 2000; updated EULAR recommendations were presented at the annual EULAR Congress in Lisbon, Portugal, in June 2003, and these have now been published.[13]

Analgesia. While acetaminophen (paracetamol) remains the first-line oral drug of choice for analgesia in patients with OA, a systemic review found that non-steroidal anti-inflammatory drugs (NSAIDs) are superior to acetaminophen for improving pain in patients with OA.[14] Furthermore, two epidemiological studies found that patients taking high doses of acetaminophen had an increased risk of upper gastrointestinal bleeding, particularly when used in combination with non-selective NSAIDs.[15,16]

The use of cyclooxygenase-2 (Cox-2) selective inhibitors in the management of patients with OA remains controversial. A systematic review of published trials showed essentially no differences in efficacy between Cox-2 selective inhibitors and traditional non-selective NSAIDs.[17] Two cost-effectiveness analyses, based on data from the large celecoxib and rofecoxib outcome

TABLE 2

Management options for osteoarthritis

Non-pharmacological

- Patient education
- Physical therapy, including aerobic and resistive exercises
- Lifestyle modification, including weight loss
- Traditional Chinese acupuncture

Pharmacological

- Nutritional supplements, including glucosamine and chondroitin sulfate
- Topical analgesics, including capsaicin and non-steroidal anti-inflammatory drugs (NSAIDs)
- Non-opioid analgesics, including acetaminophen (paracetamol)
- Oral NSAIDs, including Cox-2 selective inhibitors
- Intra-articular agents, including glucocorticoids and hyaluronate preparations
- Opioid analgesics

Surgery

- Osteotomy
- Total joint replacement

studies, concluded that Cox-2 selective inhibitors were cost-effective only in patients with a prior history of upper gastrointestinal events, including symptomatic and complicated ulcers;[18,19] one study also found that these agents were cost-effective in patients aged 75 and above even without a prior event.[18] National guidance to health professionals in the National Health Service in England and Wales states that Cox-2 selective inhibitors are not recommended for routine use in patients with OA, but should be used for the short-term management of pain in preference to standard NSAIDs when they are clearly indicated in patients at high risk of developing serious gastrointestinal adverse effects.[20]

Highlights in osteoarthritis 2003–04

WHAT'S IN?

- Use of evidence-based recommendations to guide patient management
- Recognition of the role of inflammation in disease progression
- Use of magnetic resonance imaging for evaluation of patients with painful knee osteoarthritis (OA)

WHAT'S OUT?

- Use of the terms 'degenerative joint disease' and 'osteoarthrosis'
- Routine use of arthroscopy with debridement for management of knee pain in unselected patients with knee OA

The cardiovascular safety of these agents, particularly rofecoxib, is still under scrutiny,[21,22] and more data are anticipated from ongoing clinical trials of already-marketed agents and others still in development. Because of these issues, some rheumatologists suggest that patients with OA who require anti-inflammatory agents for analgesia should take a combination of a non-selective NSAID plus a proton-pump inhibitor instead of a Cox-2 selective inhibitor, particularly if they are also on concomitant low-dose aspirin to prevent cardiovascular thrombotic events.

Disease modification and surgery. Drugs that may alter the structural progression of OA of the knee continue to be investigated in clinical trials. A pooled analysis of two randomized placebo-controlled trials of glucosamine sulfate in patients with knee OA demonstrated a statistically and clinically significant reduction in the amount of joint space narrowing over 3 years.[23] In a post-hoc analysis of data from a randomized placebo-controlled trial of sodium hyaluronate injected weekly for 3 weeks, patients with knee OA and a baseline joint-space width of 4.6 mm or greater had significantly less reduction in joint-space narrowing over 1 year than those receiving injections of saline placebo.[24] Data presented at the 2003 annual meeting of the ACR suggest that doxycycline, 100 mg twice daily, reduced the rate of joint-space narrowing compared with placebo over 30 months in overweight women with symptomatic unilateral knee OA.[25] Studies of matrix metalloprotease inhibitors, cytokine inhibitors, nitrogen-containing bisphosphonates and other agents are currently in progress and the results will be available over the next few years.

Total joint replacement remains a highly cost-effective option for patients with hip or knee OA who have moderate-to-severe pain accompanied by moderate-to-severe functional limitation. While no evidence-based recommendations for total joint replacement exist, appropriateness criteria have been developed and validated.[26,27] The National Institutes of Health convened a consensus conference in December 2003 to report on indications for and outcomes of total knee replacement in patients with OA; the statement from this conference is available from the NIH Consensus Development website.[28]

References

1. Felson DT. Osteoarthritis: new insights. Part 1: The disease and its risk factors. *Ann Intern Med* 2000; 133:637–9.

2. Pelletier J-P, Martel-Pelletier J. Osteoarthritis: from molecule to man. *Arthritis Res* 2002;4:13–19.

3. Burr DB, Radin EL. Microfractures and microcracks in subchondral bone: are they relevant to osteoarthrosis? *Rheum Dis Clin North Am* 2003;29:675–85.

4. Pelletier J-P, Martel-Pelletier J, Abramson SB. Osteoarthritis, an inflammatory disease: potential implication for the selection of new therapeutic targets. *Arthritis Rheum* 2001;44:1237–47.

5. Abramson SB, Attur M, Amin AR et al. Nitric oxide and inflammatory mediators in the perpetuation of osteoarthritis. *Curr Rheumatol Rep* 2001;3:535–41.

6. Fernandes JC, Martel-Pelletier J, Pelletier J-P. The role of cytokines in osteoarthritis pathophysiology. *Biorheology* 2002;39:237–46.

7. Raynauld JP, Kauffman C, Beaudoin G et al. Reliability of a quantification imaging system using magnetic resonance images to measure cartilage thickness and volume in human normal and osteoarthritic knees. *Osteoarthritis Cartilage* 2003;11:351–60.

8. Felson DT, Chaisson CE, Hill CL et al. The association of bone marrow lesions with pain in knee osteoarthritis. *Ann Intern Med* 2001;134:541–9.

9. Felson DT, McLaughlin S, Goggins J et al. Bone marrow edema and its relation to progression of knee osteoarthritis. *Ann Intern Med* 2003; 139:330–6.

10. Hill CL, Gale DG, Chaisson CE et al. Knee effusions, popliteal cysts, and synovial thickening: association with knee pain in osteoarthritis. *J Rheumatol* 2001;28:1330–7.

11. Hill CL, Gale DR, Chaisson CE et al. Periarticular lesions detected on magnetic resonance imaging: prevalence in knees with and without symptoms. *Arthritis Rheum* 2003;48:2836–44.

12. Felson DT. Osteoarthritis: new insights. Part 2: Treatment approaches. *Ann Intern Med* 2000;133:726–9.

13. Jordan KM, Arden NK, Doherty M et al. EULAR recommendations 2003: an evidence based approach to the management of knee osteoarthritis: Report of a Task Force of the Standing Committee for International Clinical Studies Including Therapeutic Trials (ESCISIT). *Ann Rheum Dis* 2003; 62:1145–55.

14. Towheed TE, Judd MJ, Hochberg MC et al. Acetaminophen for osteoarthritis. *Cochrane Database Sys Rev* 2003;CD004257. Oxford, Update Software (www.cochranelibrary.com).

15. Garcia Rodriguez LA, Hernandez-Diaz S. The risk of upper gastrointestinal complications associated with nonsteroidal anti-inflammatory drugs, glucocorticoids, acetaminophen and combinations of these agents. *Arthritis Res* 2001;3: 98–101.

16. Rahme E, Pettitt D, LeLorier J. Determinants and sequelae associated with utilization of acetaminophen versus traditional nonsteroidal anti-inflammatory drugs in an elderly population. *Arthritis Rheum* 2002; 46:3046–54.

17. Schnitzer TJ, Hochberg MC. COX-2 selective inhibitors in the treatment of arthritis. *Cleve Clin J Med* 2002;69:S120–30.

18. Maetzel A, Krahn M, Naglie G. The cost effectiveness of rofecoxib and celecoxib in patients with osteoarthritis or rheumatoid arthritis. *Arthritis Rheum* 2003;49:283–92.

19. Spiegel BM, Targownik L, Dulai GS et al. The cost-effectiveness of cyclooxygenase-2 selective inhibitors in the management of chronic arthritis. *Ann Intern Med* 2003;138: 795–806.

20. National Institute for Clinical Excellence. Guidance on the use of cyclo-oxygenase (Cox) II selective inhibitors, celecoxib, rofecoxib, meloxicam and etodolac for osteoarthritis and rheumatoid arthritis. *NICE Technology Appraisal Guidance* 27, 2001 (accessed at www.nice.org.uk/pdf/coxiifullguidance.pdf, December 2003).

21. Strand V, Hochberg MC. The risk of cardiovascular thrombotic events with selective cyclooxygenase-2 inhibitors. *Arthritis Rheum* 2002;47: 349–55.

22. Weir MR, Sperling RS, Reicin A et al. Selective COX-2 inhibition and cardiovascular effects: a review of the rofecoxib development program. *Am Heart J* 2003;146:591–604.

23. Richy F, Bruyere O, Ethgen O et al. Structural and symptomatic efficacy of glucosamine and chondroitin in knee osteoarthritis: a comprehensive meta-analysis. *Arch Intern Med* 2003;163:1514–22.

24. Jubb RW, Piva S, Beinat L et al. A one-year, randomised, placebo (saline) controlled clinical trial of 500-730 kDa sodium hyaluronate (Hyalgan) on the radiological change in osteoarthritis of the knee. *Int J Clin Prac* 2003;57:467–74.

25. Brandt KD, Mazzuca SA, Katz BP et al. Doxycycline slows the rate of joint space narrowing in patients with osteoarthritis. Presented at the Annual Meeting of American College of Rheumatology, October 28, 2003 (abstract LB22, accessed at www.rheumatology.org, December 2003).

26. Quintana JM, Arostegui I, Azkarate J et al. Evaluation of explicit criteria for use of total hip joint replacement. *Rheumatology* 2000;39:1234–41.

27. Escobar A, Quintana JM, Arostegui I et al. Development of explicit criteria for total knee replacement. *Int J Technol Assess Health Care* 2003;19:57–70.

28. Consensus statement from the NIH Consensus Development Conference on Total Knee Replacement, December 8–10, 2003. NIH Consensus Development Program (draft statement accessed at http://consensus.nih.gov/cons/117/117cdc_statement2.htm, December 2003).

Osteoporosis and bone

Steven R Goldring MD
Beth Israel Deaconess Medical Center, Harvard Medical School, and New England Baptist Bone and Joint Institute, Harvard Institutes of Medicine, Boston, USA

A recent National Institutes of Health (NIH) Consensus Conference on osteoporosis reviewed the epidemiological data indicating the high prevalence of osteoporosis in the general population.[1] They highlighted the devastating consequences of osteoporosis in terms of the physical, psychosocial and financial consequences, and stressed the importance of early diagnosis and attention to monitoring patients with conditions known to be associated with secondary osteoporosis. Although assessment of bone mineral density was identified as the 'gold standard' for predicting fracture risk, it was recognized that additional factors, including bone microarchitecture and quality, were also important determinants of bone strength and the ultimate risk of mechanical failure.

Epidemiological and outcome studies

Epidemiological studies indicate that more than 30% of individuals over the age of 65 have osteoporosis and are at risk for fracture. Additional investigations have highlighted the underutilization of screening techniques for diagnosing osteoporosis and the failure to initiate therapy for individuals who have sustained osteoporotic fractures.[2–4]

Solomon and co-workers analyzed the trends of osteoporosis treatment in a large cohort of elderly adults in Pennsylvania who had sustained hip or distal forearm fractures.[3] Although they found that the number of patients receiving the treatment intervention had increased steadily during the study period, by the year 2000, approximately four out of five patients who sustained a fracture were not receiving a prescription for a therapy directed at treating osteoporosis.

Additional concern regarding this issue is highlighted by a recent study reported by Kiebzak et al.[5] They reviewed the outcomes and treatment status of men and women hospitalized with hip fractures over a 5-year period. At discharge, less than 5% of the men and 27% of the women received medical therapy for osteoporosis. At 1- to 5-year follow-up, only 11% of men and 32% of women had been evaluated for osteoporosis using bone-mineral-density studies. These findings emphasize the point that osteoporosis affects males as well as females, and that the problem of underdiagnosis and lack of treatment intervention is an issue in both the female and male populations. The failure to initiate treatment in individuals with fractures is particularly troubling given that patients with prior fractures are two to five times more likely to sustain future fractures.[6] Importantly, pharmacological intervention has been shown to reduce spine and hip fracture by 40–60%.[7,8]

Glucocorticoids and bone loss
Further evidence indicating a beneficial effect of bisphosphonates on retarding glucocorticoid-induced bone loss was recently reported by Sambrook et al.[9] As documented by others, the use of bisphosphonate (alendronate) plus calcium was substantially more effective than other treatments without bisphosphonate. Among patients with inflammatory disorders, such as rheumatoid arthritis (RA), monitoring for osteoporosis and the adverse effects of glucocorticoids is of particular importance.[10,11] Patients with RA have an increased incidence of systemic osteoporosis and are at particularly high risk for fracture. This risk is increased in RA patients receiving corticosteroids.[10]

Recent studies have helped to define the mechanisms underlying the adverse effects of glucocorticoids on bone.[12] In these investigations, the authors showed that glucocorticoids depressed bone formation by inhibiting osteoblastogenesis and increasing osteoblast apoptosis. They also showed that glucocorticoids prolonged survival of osteoclasts and antagonized bisphosphonate-induced caspase activation and osteoclast apoptosis. Their findings support the hypothesis that the early rapid loss of bone induced by glucocorticoids relates to extending the lifespan of pre-existing osteoclasts. Interestingly, this early effect on osteoclast survival was not prevented by bisphosphonate treatment. Whether more aggressive treatment with higher doses of bisphosphonates or the use of more potent agents will overcome this effect warrants further investigation.

Figure 1 summarizes the regulation of bone remodeling by hormones, cytokines and therapeutic agents.

Pathogenesis of focal bone erosions in RA

Several recent studies have helped to define the role of osteoclasts in the pathogenesis of focal bone erosions in RA.[13–16] In addition to marginal joint erosions, patients with RA also have increased systemic osteoporosis.[11,17] A recent study by Schett et al. demonstrated that blockade of the receptor activator of NF-κB ligand (RANKL), which is a potent osteoclast-inducing and activating factor, with osteoprotegerin (a soluble decoy receptor for RANKL) protects against generalized bone loss in a model of inflammatory arthritis produced by overexpression of tumor necrosis factor α.[18] In a previous report, this group showed that osteoprotegerin treatment markedly inhibited the development of focal joint erosions in this animal model of arthritis.[16] These findings suggest that interfering with RANKL activity using agents such as osteoprotegerin could provide a rational strategy for preventing bone loss in inflammatory disorders as well as other forms of osteoporosis (Figure 1).

Genetic factors involved in regulating bone mass

Much has been learned in recent years about the role of genetic factors in regulating bone remodeling. Of particular interest has been the elucidation of the role of the *low-density lipoprotein receptor-related protein 5 (LRP5)* gene in regulating bone formation. *LRP5* is expressed by osteoblasts and stromal cells, and its expression is stimulated by bone morphogenic proteins. *LRP5*-null mice are osteopenic.[19] In humans, inactivating mutations of the *LRP5* gene result in decreased bone mass, and activating mutations

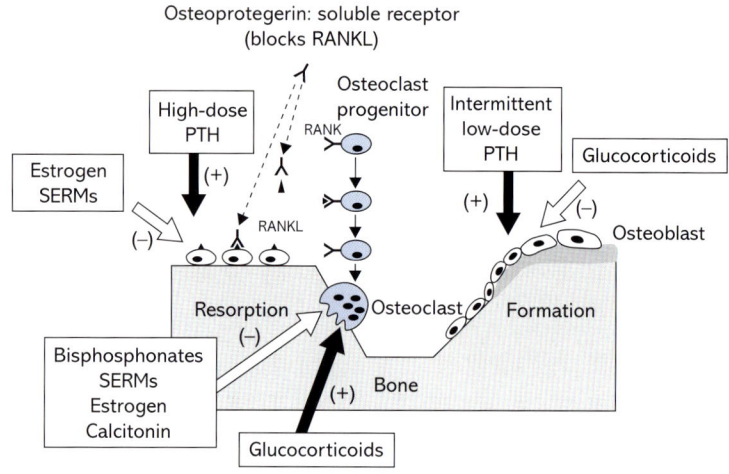

Figure 1 Regulation of bone remodeling by hormones, cytokines and therapeutic agents. Bone remodeling on trabecular bone surfaces is initiated by signals transduced by bone-lining cells. Products released by these cells, including receptor activator of NF-κB ligand (RANKL, cell surface or soluble), act through receptors (RANK) on preosteoclasts to induce osteoclast differentiation and activation. High-dose parathyroid hormone (PTH) increases RANKL expression and enhances osteoclast-mediated bone resorption. Estrogen and selective estrogen-receptor modulators (SERMs), e.g. raloxifene, suppress production of osteoclast-inducing factors. Bisphosphonates, estrogen, SERMs and calcitonin induce osteoclast apoptosis and/or decrease osteoclast activity. Glucocorticoids increase osteoclast survival. Osteoprotegerin (a RANKL decoy receptor) blocks RANKL activity. Intermittent low-dose PTH inhibits osteoblast apoptosis and increases osteoblast-mediated bone formation. Glucocorticoids induce osteoblast apoptosis and suppress bone formation.

are associated with increased bone mass.[20] More recently, Van Wesenbeeck and co-workers demonstrated the presence of missense mutations in the *LRP5* gene that were associated with several different conditions characterized by increased bone mass.[21] These results suggest that conditions with an increased bone density affecting mainly the cortices of long bones and the skull are often caused by mutations in the *LRP5* gene.

Antiresorptive therapies

Antiresorptive therapies preserve bone mass by interfering with the survival or functional activities of osteoclasts (Figure 1).[7] Their efficacy in reducing fracture incidence is related to multiple factors, including:
- the beneficial effects of reducing bone-turnover rates
- their capacity to preserve connectivity in trabecular bone
- their ability to contribute to a modest increase in bone mass (as measured by bone mineral density).[1]

These factors contribute to an improvement in bone microarchitecture and quality that ultimately translates into an increase in bone strength.

Many women using hormone replacement therapy (HRT) discontinue treatment, particularly since the publication of the results of the Women's Health Initiative that revealed the increased risk of cardiovascular complications in women taking HRT.[22] The loss of the antiresorptive bone-protective effect of estrogen exposes women to an increase in fracture risk. Methods to prevent the bone loss associated with discontinuing HRT include the use of alternative antiresorptive agents, including bisphosphonates and the selective estrogen-receptor modulator raloxifene.

In a recent study, Ascott-Evans et al. studied a group of women who had discontinued HRT.[23] They observed a high rate of bone loss in the first 12–15 months. Treatment with alendronate increased or maintained both spine and hip bone mineral density and prevented the increase in bone resorption associated with HRT withdrawal. Interestingly, in contrast to the rapid bone loss that ensues when estrogen is discontinued, women who stopped treatment with alendronate maintained bone mineral density.[24] This probably relates to the prolonged retention time of alendronate on the bone mineral surfaces resulting in sustained inhibition of osteoclast-mediated bone loss.

Anabolic agents that increase bone mass

Therapies that interfere with bone resorption have become the mainstay of osteoporosis therapy. Unfortunately, many patients do

> ## Highlights in **osteoporosis and bone** 2003–04
>
> ### WHAT'S IN?
> - Recognition that patient and physician education is needed to ensure early diagnosis and institution of therapy for osteoporosis
> - Appreciation that bone strength and resistance to fracture is determined by bone mass (as assessed by bone mineral density) **and bone quality** (indicated by history of previous fracture)
> - Antiresorptive and anabolic therapies improving bone strength by increasing bone mass and improving bone quality
> - Anabolic agents for treating osteoporosis. Intermittent parathyroid hormone increases bone mass via effects on osteoblast-mediated bone formation. Additional studies are needed to define the optimal use of combination therapy (anabolic and antiresorptive) for osteoporosis
> - The hunt for genes that regulate bone formation and resorption
>
> ### WHAT'S OUT?
> - Use of estrogen as a primary therapy for the prevention and/or treatment of osteoporosis
> - Use of bone mineral density as the sole determinant of assessing fracture risk

not come to medical attention until substantial bone loss has occurred. For this reason, there has been great interest in the development of therapeutic agents that have an anabolic effect on osteoblasts and, therefore, have the capacity to increase bone mass and improve connectivity and bone architecture.

Several recent trials have demonstrated the beneficial effects of treatment with intermittent low-dose parathyroid hormone (PTH) or a truncated recombinant form of PTH, teriparatide (recombinant human PTH 1–34) on increasing bone mass in men and women.[25-28] Although PTH is regarded as the prototypical bone-resorption-inducing hormone, paradoxically, with low-dose and intermittent administration, it preferentially increases bone mass. This effect is mediated via direct effects on osteoblasts (Figure 1).

Recent data have provided insights into the mechanisms underlying the anabolic effects of intermittent PTH. In experimental models, daily injections of PTH stimulate bone formation by attenuating osteoblast apoptosis, thereby increasing osteoblast survival, bone-formation rate and bone-mass accumulation.[29] At a molecular level, this depends on protein-kinase-A-mediated phosphorylation and inactivation of the pro-apoptotic protein Bad, as well as upregulation of survival genes such as *Bcl-2* mediated by the activation of the transcription factors cyclic AMP response element-binding protein (CREB) and runt-related transcription factor 2 (Runx2). Interestingly, when intermittent PTH is coadministered with alendronate, the anabolic effect of PTH is attenuated.[30] Although the mechanism underlying this effect needs further investigation, it could be related to the need to maintain a relatively high remodeling rate in order to provide an adequate pool of osteoblasts and osteoblast precursors to optimize the anabolic effect of intermittent PTH on bone formation. These results have important implications in terms of future approaches for combination and sequential therapies in osteoporosis. Guidelines and strategies for the use of PTH and antiresorptive agents need to be formulated.

References

1. NIH Consensus Development Panel on Osteoporosis Prevention, Diagnosis, and Therapy. Osteoporosis prevention, diagnosis, and therapy. *JAMA* 2001;285:785–95.

2. Feldstein A, Elmer P, Orwoll E et al. Bone mineral density measurement and treatment for osteoporosis in older individuals with fractures: a gap in evidence-based practice guideline implementation. *Arch Int Med* 2003;163:2165–72.

3. Solomon D, Finkelstein J, Katz J et al. Underuse of osteoporosis medications in elderly pateints with fractures. *Am J Med* 2003:115: 398–400.

4. Solomon D, Connelly M, Rosen C et al. Factors related to the use of bone densitometry: survey responses of 494 primary care physicians in New England. *Osteoporos Int* 2003;14:123–9.

5. Kiebzak G, Beinart G, Perser K et al. Undertreatment of osteoporosis in men with hip fracture. *Arch Int Med* 2002;162:2217–22.

6. Klotzbuecher C, Ross P, Landsman P et al. Patients with prior fractures have an increased risk of future fractures: a summary of the literature and statistical synthesis. *J Bone Miner Res* 2000;15:721–39.

7. Altkorn D, Vokes T. Treatment of postmenopausal osteoporosis. *JAMA* 2001;285:1415–18.

8. Drake W, Kendler D, Rosen C et al. An investigation of the predictors of bone mineral density and response to therapy with alendronate in osteoporotic men. *J Clin Endocrinol Metab* 2003;88: 5759–65.

9. Sambrook P, Kotowicz M, Nash P et al. Prevention and treatment of glucocorticoid-induced osteoporosis: a comparison of calcitriol, vitamin D plus calcium, and alendronate plus calcium. *J Bone Miner Res* 2003;18: 919–24.

10. Orstavik RE, Haugeberg G, Uhlig T et al. Vertebral deformities in 229 female patients with rheumatoid arthritis: associations with clinical variables and bone mineral density. *Arthritis Rheum* 2003;49:355–60.

11. Haugeberg G, Orstavik RE, Kvien TK. Effects of rheumatoid arthritis on bone. *Curr Opin Rheumatol* 2003;15:469–75.

12. Weinstein R, Chen J, Powers C et al. Promotion of osteoclast survival and antagonism of bisphosphonate-induced osteoclast apoptosis by glucocorticoids. *J Clin Invest* 2002;109:1041–8.

13. Pettit AR, Ji H, von Stechow D et al. TRANCE/RANKL knockout mice are protected from bone erosion in a serum transfer model of arthritis. *Am J Pathol* 2001;159:1689–99.

14. Lubberts E, Oppers-Walgreen B, Pettit AR et al. Increase in expression of receptor activator of NF-κB at sites of bone erosion correlates with progression of inflammation in evolving collagen-induced arthritis. *Arthritis Rheum* 2002;46:3055–64.

15. Redlich K, Hayer S, Ricci R et al. Osteoclasts are essential for TNF-alpha-mediated joint destruction. *J Clin Invest* 2002;110:1419–27.

16. Redlich K, Hayer S, Maier A et al. Tumor necrosis factor-α-mediated joint destruction is inhibited by targeting osteoclasts with osteoprotegerin. *Arthritis Rheum* 2002;46:785–92.

17. Goldring SR, Gravallese EM. Mechanisms of bone loss in inflammatory arthritis: diagnosis and therapeutic implications. *Arthritis Res* 2000;2:33–7.

18. Schett G, Redlich K, Hayer S et al. Osteoprotegerin protects against generalized bone loss in tumor necrosis factor-transgenic mice. *Arthritis Rheum* 2003;48:2042–51.

19. Kato M, Patel MS, Lavesseur R et al. Cbfa1-independent decrease in osteoblast proliferation, osteopenia, and persistent embryonic eye vascularization in mice deficient in Lrp5, a Wnt coreceptor. *J Cell Biol* 2002;157:303–14.

20. Boyden LM, Mao J, Belsky J et al. High bone density due to a mutation in LDL-receptor-related protein 5. *N Engl J Med* 2002;346:1513–21.

21. Van Wesenbeeck L, Cleiren E, Gram J et al. Six novel missense mutations in the LDL receptor-related protein 5 (LRP5) gene in different conditions with an increased bone density. *Am J Hum Gen* 2003;72:763–71.

22. Nelson HD, Humphrey LL, Nygren P et al. Postmenopausal hormone replacement therapy. Scientific review. *JAMA* 2002;288:872–81.

23. Ascott-Evans BH, Guanabens N, Kivinen S et al. Alendronate prevents loss of bone density associated with discontinuation of hormone replacement therapy: a randomized controlled trial. *Arch Int Med* 2003;163:789–94.

24. Greenspan SL, Emkey R, Bone HG et al. Significant differential effects of alendronate, estrogen, or combination therapy on the rate of bone loss after discontinuation of treatment of postmenopausal osteoporosis. A randomized, double-blind, placebo-controlled trial. *Ann Intern Med* 2002;137:875–83.

25. Zanchetta JR, Bogado CE, Ferretti JL et al. Effects of teriparatide [recombinant human parathyroid hormone (1-34)] on cortical bone in postmenopausal women with osteoporosis. *J Bone Miner Res* 2003;18:539–43.

26. Misof BM, Roschger P, Cosman F et al. Effects of intermittent parathyroid hormone administration on bone mineralization density in iliac crest biopsies from patients with osteoporosis: a paired study before and after treatment. *J Clin Endocrinol Metab* 2003;88:1150–6.

27. Orwoll ES, Scheele WH, Paul SR et al. The effect of teriparatide [human parathyroid (1-34)] therapy on bone density in men with osteoporosis. *J Bone Miner Res* 2003;18:9–17.

28. Finklestein JS, Hayes A, Hunzelman JL et al. The effects of parathyroid hormone, alendronate, or both in men with osteoporosis. *N Engl J Med* 2003;349:1216–26.

29. Bellido T, Ali AA, Plotkin LI et al. Proteasomal degradation of Runx2 shortens parathyroid hormone-induced anti-apoptotic signaling in osteoblasts. A putative explanation for why intermittent administration is needed for bone anabolism. *J Biol Chem* 2003;278:50259–72.

30. Black DM, Greenspan SL, Ensrud KE et al. The effects of parathyroid hormone and alendronate alone or in combination in post menopausal osteoporosis. *N Engl J Med* 2003;349:1207–15.

Systemic lupus erythematosus

Bevra H Hahn MD
David Geffen School of Medicine at UCLA, Los Angeles, California, USA

Pathogenesis

In systemic lupus erythematosus (SLE), interactions between susceptibility genes and environmental factors produce an abnormal immune response, comprising hyperactive antigen-presenting cells, T cells and B cells, resulting in autoantibody production. Some autoantibodies bind directly to target tissues, fix complement and cause damage. Other damage is mediated by immune complexes. In addition, in lupus mice, autoreactive T and B cells can cause lupus-like nephritis even in the absence of autoantibodies.

Other pathogenetic factors involve failure of the immune system to downregulate these undesirable autoreactive T and B cells, primarily by failure of control networks; immune complexes and apoptotic cells are not cleared adequately, and anti-idiotypic networks and regulatory/suppressor T cells that downregulate autoantibody production are defective. It is likely that each patient has a different combination of abnormalities that, overall, permits enough sustained autoreactivity to cause disease. As part of the abnormal response, a number of cytokines are dysregulated. For example, quantities of interferon (IFN)γ and interleukin (IL)-10 are high in peripheral blood cells or serum, whereas production of transforming growth factor (TGF)β is low. IFNγ and IL-10 both serve to drive B cells to secretion and maturation. TGFβ helps the development of regulatory/suppressive T cells.

In the past year, there has been considerable renewed interest in the cytokine type 1 IFNα, which might be a central 'boss' cytokine in SLE – similar to tumor necrosis factor α in rheumatoid arthritis. Levels of IFNα are increased in the serum of SLE patients.[1] Immune complexes containing lupus antibodies and apoptotic debris can induce the release of IFNα by plasmacytoid dendritic cells,[2] which are plentiful in biopsies of lupus skin lesions.[3] More recently, interest in this cytokine has soared because an IFN-inducible gene has been shown to be one of the major susceptibility genes in murine lupus,[4] and because several groups have shown, in the peripheral blood cells of SLE patients, a genomic 'signature' in which multiple IFNα-inducible genes are upregulated.[5–8] Real-time PCR has confirmed that the mRNA encoding some of these genes is upregulated, as is the protein product of at least one of the genes.[8] Finally, deletion of a chain of the surface receptor for type 1 IFNs protects one of the mouse models of SLE (NZB) from developing disease.[9] Biologics are in development that impair the immunostimulatory effects of IFNα, and they may be useful as therapy in SLE. On the downside, IFNα, as with type 2 IFNs (e.g. IFNγ), plays a major role in defense against viruses; non-specific interruption of this pathway is likely to predispose to infections. The immune effects of IFNα are listed in Table 1.

TABLE 1

Immune effects of the antiviral type 1 interferon (IFN) cytokine, IFNα: upregulation of the response to self

- Dendritic cells: IFNα is produced by plasmacytoid dendritic cells
- IFNα activates monocytes/macrophages
- Activated macrophages drive myeloid dendritic cells to apoptosis
- Apoptotic blebs on the surfaces of dendritic cells activate self-reactive T and B cells
- Autoreactive T and B cells together produce tissue damage, including that produced by autoantibodies
- IFNα also affects other members of the immune cell network:
    - Natural killer (NK) cells are activated: these kill other cells non-specifically
    - B cells are driven to mature and switch isotypes of Ig
    - T cells are driven to secrete interleukin (IL)-10, which increases the maturation of B cells

Therapy

Abetimus (LJP 394) is a biologic designed to 'tolerize' B cells displaying Ig surface receptors that bind DNA (i.e. B cells that secrete anti-DNA). It consists of four oligonucleotides arranged in an 'X' configuration on an inert polyethylene glycol skeleton. The idea is that the molecule binds to B-cell receptors, but does not have the capability of also binding to an Fc receptor – thus the cells receive a first signal (but not the second costimulatory signal) and become anergic rather than activated; anti-DNA production should decline. Patients who had clinically active lupus nephritis within the past 2–3 years, but were stable at the time of study entry, were randomized to receive abetimus or placebo intravenously once a week.[10] The primary outcome was time to renal flare. As predicted, in many patients, the serum levels of antibodies to double-stranded DNA fell – significantly more in the abetimus-treated group than in the control group. Time to flare, though longer in the abetimus group, did not reach statistical significance. Thus, there is proof that, in principle, this approach – a 'tolerogen' for anti-DNA B cells – can work to reduce autoantibody production. Another trial is required to demonstrate the beneficial clinical outcome.

Rituximab, an antibody to CD20, has evoked considerable interest as a potential treatment for SLE. CD20 is expressed by mature B cells; such cells are depleted by treatment with the antibody, which is approved for use in patients with certain types of B-cell lymphomas who have failed initial therapy (USA and UK). The effect does not occur in all SLE patients, however.[11] An open trial in the UK showed that a combination of high-dose corticosteroid, intravenous cyclophosphamide and rituximab led to improvement in SLE patients with severe disease refractory to standard therapies.[12] It is likely that additional studies will establish the role of this biologic in SLE.

Cyclophosphamide regimens. Another European study challenged the standard 'National Institutes for Health (NIH) regimen' for cyclophosphamide treatment.[13] Lower doses of cyclophosphamide were compared with standard doses in patients with active lupus nephritis. One group received the NIH cyclophosphamide regimen, beginning at 500 mg/m^2 monthly and escalating to doses required to cause leukopenia. It was given for 6 months, followed by two more doses at 3-monthly intervals. The other group received cyclophosphamide, 500 mg i.v. every 2 weeks for six doses. Both groups at the conclusion of cyclophosphamide therapy were maintained on azathioprine. Initial treatment included intravenous pulsed corticosteroid, followed by a daily oral dose of 0.5 mg/kg prednisolone. A response rate of approximately 80% was achieved in both groups. There were fewer episodes of infection in the low-dose group, but the difference did not achieve statistical significance. Therefore, a cumulative dose of 3 g cyclophosphamide may be as beneficial as the much higher dose (approximately 8 g/year) given in the NIH regimen. Most patients were followed for only 12 months. It is well known that the benefits of various treatments for lupus nephritis may not be sustained, and differences may require 4–5 years to be detectable. Patients in this trial were primarily Caucasian; the milder therapy may be less successful in ethnic groups in whom lupus nephritis has a worse outcome, such as African Americans and mestizo-background Hispanics. Nevertheless, the study raises the important question of what is the best dose and administration regimen for cyclophosphamide in patients with active, severe SLE.

Mycophenolate mofetil. Finally, a study presented recently in abstract form has suggested that mycophenolate mofetil may be as good as, and safer than, cyclophosphamide therapy in the management of lupus nephritis.[14] A previous study of patients with lupus nephritis from Hong Kong showed equivalent responses to daily mycophenolate mofetil and oral cyclophosphamide (2–3 mg/kg/day) for 6 months followed by azathioprine.[15] The duration of that study was 12 months. In the recent study, US patients with active lupus nephritis were randomized to receive the NIH cyclophosphamide regimen (described above), or mycophenolate mofetil in escalating doses reaching 3 g daily.[14]

Highlights in **systemic lupus erythematosus** 2003–04

WHAT'S IN?

- Interferon (IFN)α as a potential central 'boss' cytokine in autoreactivity
- A genomic 'signature' from peripheral blood cells of SLE patients, which includes upregulation of several genes controlled by type 1 and type 2 IFNs
- Mycophenolate mofetil as a potential inducer of remission for lupus nephritis
- Abetimus (LJP 394) as a biologic that reduces serum levels of anti-DNA antibodies (not available for use)
- Topical tacrolimus for lupus skin rash[16]
- Thalidomide for non-responsive skin rashes[17]

WHAT'S OUT?

- Recommending induction of remission with high-dose cyclophosphamide without considering alternatives depending on disease features and ethnicity of the patient
- Considering maintaining improvement with many months of quarterly cyclophosphamide without considering alternatives depending on degree of response to induction therapy, disease features and ethnicity of the patient

The duration of the study was 6 months. The proportion of patients who improved was significantly higher in the mycophenolate mofetil group. The infection rate was lower with mycophenolate mofetil, but gastrointestinal side effects, particularly diarrhea, were more frequent.

Treatment of severe lupus dermatitis. Recently, several groups have reported open trials of topical tacrolimus, and systemic thalidomide in the management of severe dermatitis (particularly the rashes of systemic lupus or subacute cutaneous lupus).[16,17] Topical tacrolimus can replace high-to-moderate-intensity topical corticosteroids in some patients, thus reducing the chance of skin atrophy. For more severe dermatitis, thalidomide at doses from 50 mg every other day to 100 mg daily for a few weeks produces improvement in most patients who have failed traditional treatments. Most experts consider thalidomide an advance in therapeutics, but its use is constrained by adverse effects that include extreme teratogenicity, drowsiness (with a high prevalence), and peripheral neuropathies that are sometimes irreversible.

References

1. Hooks JJ, Moutsopoulos HM, Geis SA et al. Immune interferon in the circulation of patients with autoimmune diseases. *N Engl J Med* 1979;301:5–8.

2. Blomberg S, Elorant J-L, Magnusson M et al. Expression of the markers BDCA-2 and BCDA-4 and production of interferon-α by plasmacytoid dendritic cells in SLE. *Arthritis Rheum* 2003;48:2524–32.

3. Bave U, Alm GV, Ronnblom L. The combination of apoptotic U937 cells and lupus IgG is a potent IFN-α inducer. *J Immunol* 2000;165:3519–26.

4. Rozzo SJ, Allard JD, Choubey D et al. Evidence for an interferon-inducible gene Ifi202, in the susceptibility to systemic lupus. *Immunity* 2001;15:435–43.

5. Crow MK. Interferon-α: a new target for therapy in SLE. *Arthritis Rheum* 2003;48:2396–401.

6. Baechler EC, Batliwalla FM, Karypis G et al. Interferon-inducible gene expression signature in peripheral blood cells of patients with severe lupus. *Proc Natl Acad Sci USA* 2003;100:2610–5.

7. Bennett L, Palucka AK, Arce E et al. Interferon and granulopoiesis signatures in systemic lupus erythematosus blood. *J Exp Med* 2003;197:711–23.

8. Ye S, Pang H, Gu YY et al. Protein interaction for an interferon-inducible systemic lupus associated gene, IFIT1. *Rheumatology (Oxford)* 2003;42:1155–63.

9. Santiago-Raber ML, Baccala R, Haraldsson KM et al. Type-I interferon receptor deficiency reduces lupus-like disease in NZB mice. *J Exp Med* 2003;197:777–88.

10. Alarcon-Segovia D, Tumlin JA, Furie RA et al. LJP 394 Investigator Consortium. LJP 394 for the prevention of renal flare in patients with systemic lupus erythematosus: results from a randomized, double-blind, placebo-controlled study. *Arthritis Rheum* 2003;48:442–54.

11. Anolik J, Campbell D, Felgar RE et al. The relationship of Fcgamma RIIIA genotype to degree of B cell depletion by rituximab in the treatment of systemic lupus erythematosus. *Arthritis Rheum* 2003:48:455–9.

12. Leandro MJ, Edwards JC, Cambridge G et al. An open study of B lymphocyte depletion in systemic lupus erythematosus. *Arthritis Rheum* 2002;46:2673–7.

13. Houssiau FA, Vasconcelos C, D'Cruz D et al. Immunosuppressive therapy in lupus nephritis: the Euro-Lupus Nephritis Trial, a randomized trial of low-dose versus high-dose intravenous cyclophosphamide. *Arthritis Rheum* 2002:46:2121–31.

14. Ginzler EM, Aranow C, Buyon J et al. A multicenter study of mycophenolate mofetil (MMF) vs intravenous cyclophosphamide (IVC) as induction therapy for severe lupus nephritis (LN): preliminary results. *Arthritis Rheum* 2003;48:S647.

15. Chan TM, Li FK, Tang CS et al. Efficacy of mycophenolate mofetil in patients with diffuse proliferative lupus nephritis. Hong Kong-Guangzhou Nephrology Study Group. *N Engl J Med* 2000;343: 1156–62.

16. Callen JP. Management of skin disease in patients with lupus erythematosus. *Best Pract Res Clin Rheumatol* 2002;16:245–64.

17. Pelle MT, Werth VP. Thalidomide in cutaneous lupus erythematosus. *Am J Clin Dermatol* 2003;4:379–87.

Scleroderma

Christopher P Denton PhD FRCP
Centre for Rheumatology, Royal Free Hospital, London, UK

Scleroderma (systemic sclerosis, SSc) is a prototypic multisystem connective-tissue disease that has a substantial mortality compared with other autoimmune rheumatic diseases. It is heterogeneous, with two major subsets: limited cutaneous and diffuse cutaneous SSc. Subset differentiation is based on the presence and absence of proximal limb and truncal skin involvement. The subsets themselves are heterogeneous with respect to the pattern and extent of internal organ involvement, and severity of skin sclerosis. Two other less frequent subsets are systemic sclerosis sine scleroderma and limited SSc.

Systemic sclerosis sine scleroderma has the vascular and internal organ complications of SSc without apparent skin involvement.[1] Patients with this invariably have an SSc hallmark autoantibody.

The designation of limited SSc as a category is not yet universally accepted as this category overlaps with that formerly termed autoimmune Raynaud's phenomenon. Patients have an SSc hallmark antibody, Raynaud's phenomenon and the characteristic SSc nailfold capillaroscopic abnormalities.[2] They lack skin sclerosis and major organ-based complications. The natural history of this group remains uncertain.

Risk stratification

Ultimately, modern approaches to scleroderma genetics are likely to identify susceptibility and severity genes. New approaches include gene-profiling experiments, which have so far identified over- and underexpressed genes associated with lesional scleroderma skin and fibroblasts. Interestingly, many of these genes are regulated by transforming growth factor (TGF)β, providing additional evidence that this is a key growth factor in the pathogenesis of SSc.[3]

Association studies include a recent genome-wide screen of Choctaw Native American patients.[4] There has been recent interest in comparing gene expression in non-involved skin sites with expression in healthy controls to determine potential susceptibility loci.[5]

Serological associations are now much better understood. It has been clearly shown that the ability of an individual to respond to immunogenic determinants of hallmark SSc autoantigens is associated with certain class II human leukocyte antigen (HLA) alleles. This is consistent with current understanding of antigen presentation and accessory/costimulatory signals. It is less certain whether such associations are held across different ethnic or geographic boundaries, though an ongoing study in three different North American groups is expected to address these issues specifically.[6]

Within single-center cohorts, associations are now well established (Table 1). It appears that anti-RNA polymerase I or III reactivity is an independent risk factor for scleroderma renal crisis, though anti-topoisomerase-1 is not. There is increased frequency of anti-topoisomerase-1 with interstitial pulmonary fibrosis. Anti-fibrillarin (also termed U3-ribonucleoprotein) reactivity is associated with a poor outcome, particularly in diffuse cutaneous SSc.[7]

Pulmonary hypertension occurs commonly in SSc. It is associated with anti-centromere-antibody reactivity and also with anti-fibrillarin reactivity. In the latter, it occurs typically in the absence of major lung fibrosis. Ultimately, serologically defined subsets may be helpful in risk stratification when used in conjunction with other clinical features, so that protocols for investigating, monitoring and treating SSc patients can be individualized. Eventually, genetic markers and other soluble serum factors are likely to be used in a similar way.[8]

Pathogenesis

The multifaceted nature of the pathogenesis of SSc has now become more clearly understood. The interplay between the vascular, inflammatory and fibrotic processes is appreciated and a number of

TABLE 1

Clinical associations of hallmark autoantibodies in systemic sclerosis (SSc)

Autoantibody reactivity	Clinical association
Centromere (ACA)	• Limited cutaneous SSc • Isolated pulmonary arterial hypertension • Bad gut disease
Topoisomerase-1 (Scl-70)	• Lung fibrosis • Diffuse cutaneous SSc • Renal crisis
RNApol I, III	• Renal disease • Diffuse cutaneous SSc (additional risk factor for renal crisis through independent association of this antibody with diffuse skin disease)
Fibrillarin (U3-RNP)	• Pulmonary hypertension • Myositis • Renal crisis
Pm-Scl	• Polymyositis • Lung fibrosis
U1-RNP	• Overlap features of systemic lupus erythematosus • Polymyositis • Arthritis
Th/To	• Pulmonary hypertension in limited cutaneous SSc

potentially important mediators of intercellular cross-talk have been identified (Figure 1). In time, these will suggest logical target factors or signaling pathways for therapeutic intervention.

The ultimate effector cells of scleroderma are matrix-synthesizing fibroblastic cells. These often express the markers and phenotypic properties of myofibroblasts.[9] Evidence suggests that there may be phenotypic fluidity between fibroblasts and myofibroblasts, and between vasculature components such as microvascular pericytes. It has also been suggested that circulating progenitor cells may be deposited at sites of fibrosis. As a corollary, circulating endothelial cells have recently been reported, though

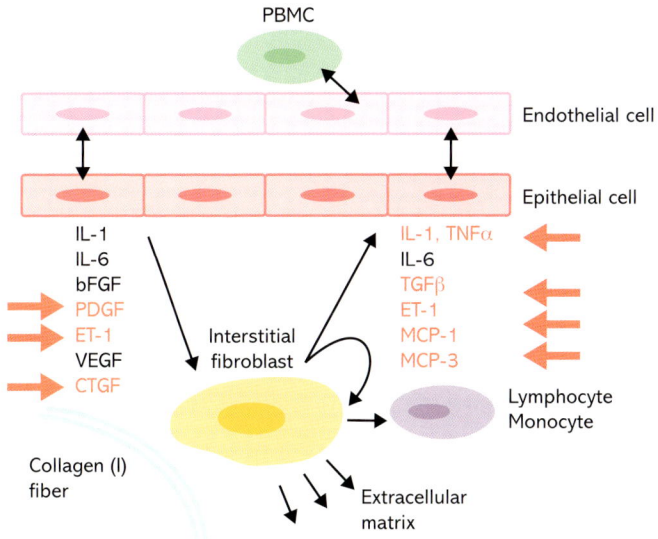

Figure 1 Targeting intercellular cross-talk in scleroderma. The pathogenesis of scleroderma involves initial vascular events that lead to the activation of perivascular fibroblasts and transient but marked interstitial inflammation with mononuclear inflammatory cells. Epithelial damage may be equally important in organs such as the lung, gut and kidney in which there is extensive juxtaposition of epithelial and endothelial cell layers. Each cell type produces a range of cytokine mediators that modulate the properties of other cell types, and the ultimate persistence of a fibrotic phenotype for fibroblasts reflects a mature cytokine network. It is theoretically possible to interrupt this at a number of levels (red arrows) with currently available drugs including endothelin-receptor antagonists and agents blocking tumor necrosis factor (TNF)α. Other putative targets include chemokine (MCP-1, -3) receptors, connective tissue growth factor (CTGF) and transforming growth factor (TGF)β. Some of these agents are currently in clinical trials or in preclinical development. PBMC, peripheral blood mononuclear cell; IL, interleukin; bFGF, basic fibroblast growth factor; PDGF, platelet-derived growth factor; ET-1, endothelin-1; VEGF, vascular endothelial growth factor; MCP, monocyte chemotactic protein.

these studies remain preliminary. Embryonically defined regulatory elements within extracellular-matrix genes have recently been identified as potential targets for activation in a mouse model of scleroderma and these elements are also present in human matrix genes. That there could be a persistent population of cells in which embryonically defined pathways of gene regulation are active and can be upregulated is intriguing. It suggests that there may be a resident population of progenitor fibroblasts that can be activated in fibrosis.[10]

Assessing skin involvement

Skin sclerosis is the hallmark clinical feature of most cases of SSc and it remains the clinical manifestation that mostly commonly triggers a correct diagnosis. The Rodnan skin score, originally a cumbersome and complex clinical tool, has now been developed and refined. It is now well validated, with scores being shown to associate with outcome and organ-based complications in SSc.[11]

Other methods of assessing skin involvement have also been tested. A suction device measured skin involvement reproducibly in a cross-sectional study.[12] Interestingly, there were abnormal skin biomechanics even in clinically normal sites. This suggests either a much more widespread pathology even in limited cutaneous SSc, or systemic differences in connective tissue. The latter might imply that susceptibility to or severity of SSc is genetically determined. An altered fibrillin metabolism that is apparently genetically determined has been reported in patients with SSc,[13] and this may provide a mechanism that explains altered vascular biomechanics in SSc. This finding could have implications for larger vessel disease in SSc.[14] Another device that has been developed to test skin biomechanics applies torsional forces.[15] A device measuring skin hardness (a durometer) is also being tested.

Assessing clinical impact

The scleroderma health-assessment questionnaire (SHAQ) is now in common clinical use, but the simpler SSc functional score has been shown to be associated with individual visual-analog scale components of the SHAQ.[16] Organ-specific questionnaires are also being developed. Severity and activity initiatives are under way.

Scleroderma-associated lung disease

Pulmonary complications are the main cause of SSc-associated death. A multifaceted approach to investigation is necessary, involving symptom assessment, pulmonary function tests (PFTs), high-resolution computed tomography (HRCT), bronchoalveolar lavage and nebulized radionuclide (DTPA) lung scanning. Longitudinal studies suggest that PFTs are predictive of progression, but only after a follow-up period of up to 3 years. HRCT images can be readily quantified using simple validated scoring systems.

In SSc, non-specific interstitial pneumonia (NSIP) histology predominates, in contrast to the findings in patients with idiopathic pulmonary fibrosis. NSIP histology can now be readily distinguished from usual interstitial pneumonia by HRCT.[17] Interestingly, the histological pattern does not predict outcome, though this may reflect the small number of patients with the histological pattern of usual interstitial pneumonia or the effect of treatment or follow-up bias determined by the subtype of clinical features.[18] This is in contrast to what is seen in idiopathic pulmonary fibrosis. There have been many studies suggesting that cyclophosphamide, given orally or by intravenous infusion, is beneficial in SSc. However, these have often been retrospective and hence poorly controlled. A recent small prospective series was encouraging, suggesting stabilization of lung fibrosis in SSc.[19] Clinical trials are under way that should address the value of cyclophosphamide. It is likely, however, that investigational features and clinical context also need to be taken into consideration when identifying patients most likely to benefit from this agent. Bosentan (see later) is currently being tried for SSc-associated as well as idiopathic pulmonary fibrosis.

Pulmonary arterial hypertension

Pulmonary arterial hypertension occurs in approximately 8% of patients with SSc and has a high mortality.[20,21] Its association with connective tissue diseases, particularly SSc, is now well established. It can develop as an isolated complication or secondary to pulmonary fibrosis. It has also been suggested that pulmonary vascular disease can occur in SSc without necessarily progressing to hemodynamically significant pulmonary hypertension.[22]

There have been significant advances in assessment and therapy for pulmonary arterial hypertension, and there are now well-established diagnostic criteria. On right heart catheterization, resting mean pulmonary artery pressure above 25 mmHg or greater than 30 mmHg during exercise are diagnostic. Clinical features and simple investigations such as echocardiography, Doppler echocardiography and PFTs are useful and also assist with important differential diagnoses, such as cardiac involvement or interstitial lung fibrosis. Other causes of pulmonary hypertension must be excluded and radioisotope ventilation:perfusion scans and CT pulmonary angiography are important, the latter being particularly useful in patients with associated interstitial lung disease that complicates ventilation. Additional cardiac tests might also be needed to exclude coronary arterial or intrinsic cardiac disease. Inflammatory myocarditis is often associated with elevated cardiac-specific creatine kinase (CKMB) and troponin levels. Gated cardiac magnetic resonance imaging (MRI) appears to be a valuable research tool that may be applied when diagnosing both cardiac and pulmonary vascular disease through its effects on the cardiac cavity, and muscle mass and movement.

Drawing from experience of primary pulmonary hypertension, treating this complication in the context of SSc is now possible. Patients should receive oral anticoagulation and oxygen supplementation. Calcium-channel blockers are rarely effective, but parenteral prostacyclin analogs improve functional capacity and pulmonary hemodynamics. The oral endothelin-receptor blocker bosentan has now also been shown to be an effective therapy for established symptomatic pulmonary hypertension in SSc.[23] Oxygen is useful for exertional dyspnea, and long-term (16 hours/day) low-flow oxygen via nasal specula can be used with the aim of reducing or reversing hypoxia-induced pulmonary vasoconstriction.

Other important potential problems associated with using continuous intravenous prostacyclin for pulmonary arterial hypertension include line sepsis, the catastrophic effect of pump failure following acute withdrawal of prostanoids in established patients, and the general problems of long-term ambulatory central venous catheterization.[24]

Cardiac disease

The stress of intercurrent illness, sepsis, fluid load or electrolyte disturbance seem to be important triggers for cardiac manifestations of SSc.[25] Cardiac involvement in scleroderma is variable in severity and clinical significance. Patients may develop fibrosis of the myocardium or conducting tissue, leading to impaired biventricular function and hemodynamically significant arrhythmias including heart block. Inflammatory myocarditis is uncommon, but warrants intervention with immunosuppressive treatment when associated with impaired left ventricular function. Pericardial disease with effusion is frequent, but rarely hemodynamically compromising; specific intervention is generally unnecessary.

Although major cardiac involvement can be detected by simple tests such as echocardiography (including stress-echo), it may be underestimated by long-term electrocardiographic monitoring and nuclear-medicine evaluation of cardiac output and focal myocardial function. Gated cardiac MRI has proven useful in determining the structure and function of the right and left heart chambers, and is probably the most discriminating test, though at present it is largely confined to use as a research tool.

It seems that patients with scleroderma may have occult left ventricular cardiac involvement that can become more of a problem at times of cardiovascular stress related to the disease (e.g. hypertensive renal crisis) or to therapies associated with high volume fluid loads, or as a result of cardiotoxic drugs (e.g. marrow-ablative doses of cyclophosphamide).[26] Right ventricular failure appears to be the main determinant of mortality in scleroderma-associated pulmonary hypertension, and the long-term effectiveness of advanced therapies for pulmonary

Highlights in scleroderma 2003–04

WHAT'S IN?
- Regular screening for organ-based complications
- Early right heart catheterization and advanced therapies for suspected pulmonary arterial hypertension
- Integration of tests to detect early pulmonary disease
- Risk stratification by subset, stage and antinuclear antibody reactivity
- Endothelin-receptor blockade as potential disease-modifying therapy

WHAT'S OUT?
- Limited cutaneous systemic sclerosis (SSc) as a benign disease
- Scl-70 as a marker only of diffuse cutaneous SSc
- Idiopathic pulmonary fibrosis as a model for SSc-associated lung fibrosis

hypertension will depend on their ability to stabilize or improve indices of right ventricular function.

Renal disease

It is now appreciated that there is often a background impairment in renal function, with reduced glomerular filtration rate compared with matched healthy controls.[27] This may reflect interstitial fibrosis or subclinical vasculopathy. Although angiotensin-converting enzyme (ACE) inhibitors remain the mainstay of treating established hypertensive renal crises in scleroderma, it is possible that additional therapy (e.g. with angiotensin-receptor blockers) may also be helpful. This needs to be addressed in clinical trials. A recent population-based study has confirmed that hypertensive renal crisis occurs in patients with limited cutaneous SSc as well those with diffuse cutaneous SSc, albeit with substantially lower frequency.[28]

References

1. Poormoghim H, Lucas M, Fertig N et al. Systemic sclerosis sine scleroderma: demographic, clinical, and serologic features and survival in forty-eight patients. *Arthritis Rheum* 2000;43:444–51.

2. LeRoy EC, Medsger TA Jr. Criteria for the classification of early systemic sclerosis. *J Rheumatol* 2001;28:1573–6.

3. Ahmed SS, Tan FK. Identification of novel targets in scleroderma: update on population studies, cDNA arrays, SNP analysis, and mutations. *Curr Opin Rheumatol* 2003;15:766–71.

4. Zhou X, Tan FK, Wang N et al. Genome-wide association study for regions of systemic sclerosis susceptibility in a Choctaw Indian population with high disease prevalence. *Arthritis Rheum* 2003;48:2585–92.

5. Whitfield ML, Finlay DR, Murray JI et al. Systemic and cell type-specific gene expression patterns in scleroderma skin. *Proc Natl Acad Sci USA* 2003;100:12319–24.

6. Reveille JD, Fischbach M, McNearney T et al. GENISOS Study Group. Systemic sclerosis in 3 US ethnic groups: a comparison of clinical, sociodemographic, serologic, and immunogenetic determinants. *Semin Arthritis Rheum* 2001;30:332–46.

7. Bunn CC, Denton CP, Shi-Wen X et al. Anti-RNA polymerases and other autoantibody specificities in systemic sclerosis. *Br J Rheumatol* 1998;37:15–20.

8. Tormey VJ, Bunn CC, Denton CP, Black CM. Anti-fibrillarin antibodies in systemic sclerosis. *Rheumatology* 2001;40:1157–62.

9. Kissin E, Korn JH. Apoptosis and myofibroblasts in the pathogenesis of systemic sclerosis. *Curr Rheumatol Rep* 2002;4:129–35.

10. Denton CP, Zheng B, Shiwen X et al. Activation of a fibroblast-specific enhancer of the proα2(I) collagen gene in tight-skin mice. *Arthritis Rheum* 2001;44:712–22.

11. DeMarco PJ, Weisman MH, Seibold JR et al. Predictors and outcomes of scleroderma renal crisis: the high-dose versus low-dose D-penicillamine in early diffuse systemic sclerosis trial. *Arthritis Rheum* 2002;46:2983–9.

12. Balbir-Gurman A, Denton CP, Nichols B et al. Non-invasive measurement of biomechanical skin properties in systemic sclerosis. *Ann Rheum Dis* 2002;61:237–41.

13. Wallis DD, Tan FK, Kielty CM et al. Abnormalities in fibrillin 1-containing microfibrils in dermal fibroblast cultures from patients with systemic sclerosis (scleroderma). *Arthritis Rheum* 2001;44:1855–64.

14. Cheng KS, Tiwari A, Boutin A et al. Carotid and femoral arterial wall mechanics in scleroderma. *Rheumatology* 2003;42:1299–305.

15. Knight LR, Smeathers JE, Isdale AH et al. Evaluating the cutaneous involvement in scleroderma: torsional stiffness revisited. *Rheumatology* 2001;40:128–32.

16. Smyth AE, MacGregor AJ, Mukerjee D et al. A cross-sectional comparison of three self-reported functional indices in scleroderma. *Rheumatology* 2003;42:732–8.

17. Desai SR, Veeraraghavan S, Hansell DM et al. CT features of interstitial lung disease in systemic sclerosis, usual interstitial pneumonitis and non-specific interstitial pneumonitis. *Radiology*, in press.

18. Bouros D, Wells AU, Nicholson AG et al. Histopathologic subsets of fibrosing alveolitis in patients with systemic sclerosis and their relationship to outcome. *Am J Respir Crit Care Med* 2002;165:1581–6.

19. Griffiths B, Miles S, Moss H et al. Systemic sclerosis and interstitial lung disease: a pilot study using pulse intravenous methylprednisolone and cyclophosphamide to assess the effect on high resolution computed tomography scan and lung function. *J Rheumatol* 2002;29:2371–8.

20. Mukerjee D, St George D, Coleiro B et al. Prevalence and outcome in systemic sclerosis associated pulmonary arterial hypertension: application of a registry approach. *Ann Rheum Dis* 2003;62:1088–93.

21. Kawut SM, Taichman DB, Archer-Chicko CL et al. Hemodynamics and survival in patients with pulmonary arterial hypertension related to systemic sclerosis. *Chest* 2003;123:344–50.

22. Denton CP, Black CM. Pulmonary hypertension in systemic sclerosis. *Rheum Dis Clin North Am* 2003;29:335–49.

23. Rubin LJ, Badesch DB, Barst RJ et al. Bosentan therapy for pulmonary arterial hypertension. *N Engl J Med* 2002;346:896–903.

24. British Cardiac Society Guidelines and Medical Practice Committee, and approved by the British Thoracic Society and the British Society of Rheumatology. Recommendations on the management of pulmonary hypertension in clinical practice. *Heart* 2001;86:11–13.

25. Coghlan JG, Mukerjee D. The heart and pulmonary vasculature in scleroderma: clinical features and pathobiology. *Curr Opin Rheumatol* 2001;13:495–9.

26. Van Laar JM, Tyndall A. Intense immunosuppression and stem-cell transplantation for patients with severe rheumatic autoimmune disease: a review. *Cancer Control* 2003;10:57–65.

27. Kingdon EJ, Knight CJ, Dustan K et al. Calculated glomerular filtration rate is a useful screening tool to identify scleroderma patients with renal impairment. *Rheumatology* 2003;42:26–33.

28. Hesselstrand R, Scheja A, Shen GQ et al. The association of antinuclear antibodies with organ involvement and survival in systemic sclerosis. *Rheumatology* 2003;42:534–40.

Vasculitis treatment

David Jayne MD FRCP
Vasculitis and Lupus Clinic, Addenbrooke's Hospital, Cambridge, UK

Vasculitis occurs as a localized or systemic process. It may be a primary disorder or result from an identifiable cause, such as a drug, an infection or malignancy. The major subgroup of primary systemic vasculitis is the small vessel vasculitides with few or absent immune deposits and circulating autoantibodies to neutrophil cytoplasmic antigens (ANCA, 'ANCA-associated vasculitis'). This group includes Wegener's granulomatosis, microscopic polyangiitis and Churg–Strauss angiitis. The clinical presentations are heterogeneous, with some clinical features common to more than one syndrome. The treatment principles are similar across the group. The advent of combination prednisolone and cyclophosphamide therapy in the 1970s heralded a major advance in vasculitis treatment and this remains the gold standard against which newer approaches are compared.

A subclassification of systemic vasculitis by disease severity at presentation is shown in Table 1. Patients without an imminent threat to vital organ function are classified as having early systemic disease. Treatment with oral prednisolone and weekly methotrexate is as effective for the induction of remission as prednisolone and daily oral cyclophosphamide.[1]

For those with threatened vital organ function, including renal vasculitis, prednisolone and cyclophosphamide are employed until remission occurs, usually between 3 and 6 months.[2] It is then safe to withdraw cyclophosphamide and introduce either azathioprine or methotrexate. This approach minimizes the risk of hemorrhagic cystitis, bladder cancer and myeloproliferative disorders previously observed in vasculitis patients undergoing long-term cyclophosphamide therapy.

TABLE 1

Classification of vasculitis at diagnosis according to disease severity

Clinical subgroup	Constitutional symptoms	Typical ANCA status	Threatened vital organ function	Serum creatinine (µmol/liter)
Localized	No	Positive or negative	No	< 120
Early systemic	Yes	Positive	No	< 120
Generalized	Yes	Positive	Yes	< 500
Severe renal	Yes	Positive	Yes	> 500
Refractory	Yes	Positive or negative	Yes	Any

ANCA, autoantibodies to neutrophil cytoplasmic antigens

Controversy exists as to whether intravenous pulsed cyclophosphamide is superior to daily oral administration, with the former being safer but associated with a higher risk of relapse.[3] Pulsed regimens have varied in dose and dosing interval: the consensus regimen of the European Vasculitis Study Group employs a dose of 15 mg/kg with an initial 2-week interval lengthening to a 3-week interval after the third dose (see www.vasculitis.org). Fulminant presentations with vital organ failure, including rapidly progressive glomerulonephritis and pulmonary hemorrhage, receive additional therapy with pulsed methylprednisolone or plasma exchange.[4]

Polyarteritis nodosa predominantly involves muscular arteries, and prognostic factors at diagnosis have been determined.[5] In those with at least one adverse prognostic factor, a 12-month course of monthly pulsed cyclophosphamide has proved superior to a shorter course for both rates of remission and relapse.[6]

Disease monitoring and relapse

Disease activity in ANCA-associated vasculitis is monitored by clinical assessment and the serological variables, C-reactive protein

(CRP), erythrocyte sedimentation rate (ESR) and ANCA. Both CRP and ESR are influenced by intercurrent infection and ANCA levels do not correlate well with disease activity while patients are on immunosuppressive therapy. The real value of ANCA in monitoring vasculitis is during reduction or withdrawal of therapy, when a persistently positive or markedly rising ANCA level is strongly predictive of subsequent relapse.[7] Clinical assessments of disease activity and damage have been standardized by the Birmingham Vasculitis Activity Score (BVAS) and Vasculitis Damage Index (VDI).[8] These tools have prognostic value for therapeutic responses and disease outcomes, provide a method for recording the extent and severity of disease and serve as endpoints for clinical trials.

Primary treatment failure is uncommon, though up to 50% of patients experience a disease relapse, usually as treatment is reduced or withdrawn.[2,9] Relapse is more common in Wegener's granulomatosis and in those with persistent ANCA positivity, and less common in those with renal involvement.[10] Remission maintenance protocols employ either azathioprine or methotrexate with or without low-dose prednisolone. Over one-third of those on methotrexate relapse within 20 months, often after steroid withdrawal.[11] The optimal duration of remission maintenance therapy is unclear; it should probably be prolonged for those with Wegener's granulomatosis, persisting ANCA positivity or a previous history of relapse. Ongoing clinical trials are comparing regimens of 2 and 4 years' duration, and azathioprine with methotrexate and mycophenolate mofetil.[4]

Frequently relapsing patients or those with incomplete disease control have refractory vasculitis. They are at high risk of irreversible drug toxicity. There is no consensus on their optimal management but typically they receive further courses of cyclophosphamide or alternative immunosuppressive drugs, such as mycophenolate mofetil or leflunomide. High-dose intravenous immunoglobulin has an antivasculitic effect but is expensive and needs to be repeated at 1- to 3-month intervals.[12] Infection often plays a role in relapse in Wegener's granulomatosis, and long-term co-trimoxazole reduces relapse rates.[13] More recently, nasal mupirocin ointment has been evaluated in this indication.[14]

Toxicity

Current induction protocols lead to severe adverse events in 25% of patients and these are more frequent with severe disease, older age and renal impairment.[1,9] Cyclophosphamide doses should be reduced for age and renal impairment, and leukopenia avoided because it relates directly to septic death.[9] Infection remains the major cause of death but its frequency can be minimized by careful monitoring of the white-blood-cell count, with cyclophosphamide being reduced or withdrawn before leukopenia occurs. Current corticosteroid doses remain high (initial prednisolone dose 1 mg/kg/day), though recent protocols are tapering the dose more quickly and allowing early withdrawal.[11] The use of prophylaxis against *Pneumocystis carinii* pneumonia, fungal infections, peptic ulceration and steroid-induced bone disease has become routine based on the high frequency of these complications in the past.[14] Despite these precautions, reduction of treatment toxicity is the major incentive for newer therapeutic approaches.

Outcome

The risks of death and end-stage renal failure are related to age and serum creatinine; disease subgrouping at diagnosis strongly predicts outcome (Figure 1).[1,5,9] Renal histology is predictive of renal outcome, with acute lesions (including cellular crescents and necrotic foci) being positively related with outcome. Fibrotic changes predict a poorer outcome. Non-healing scars of disease are often already present at diagnosis, and further items accrue as a consequence of vasculitic inflammation, drug toxicity or intercurrent disease.[2,8] The patient's functional status is severely impaired at diagnosis, and remains significantly below that of healthy comparators during the remission phase.[2] This aspect of vasculitis is a major contributor to morbidity and is incompletely understood. It may reflect poor rehabilitation, ongoing subclinical disease, drug toxicity or the consequences of previous damage.

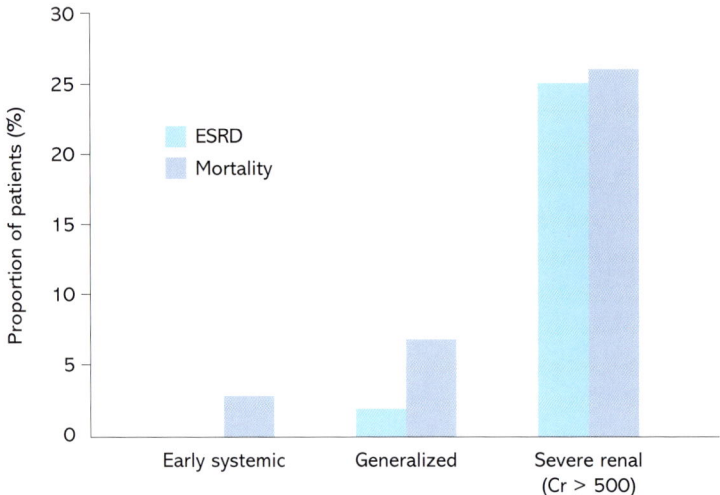

Figure 1 One-year outcome according to mortality and end-stage renal disease (ESRD) for early systemic disease, generalized disease and severe renal vasculitis. Cr > 500 indicates serum creatinine > 500 µmol/liter. Reproduced with permission from S Karger AG, Basel.[1]

The newer agents

T-cell depletion with either antithymocyte globulin or alemtuzumab has been effective in refractory vasculitis and has led to prolonged treatment-free remissions, but toxicity limits widespread use.[15,16] Results of preliminary studies with tumor necrosis factor (TNF)α blockade by infliximab and etanercept are exciting and this approach has the potential to be steroid-sparing and induce more rapid remissions.[17,18] Alternative immunosuppressive agents, including leflunomide, ciclosporin, mycophenolate mofetil and gusperimus (deoxyspergualin), have shown efficacy in open-label studies.[19] B-cell depletion with rituximab is attracting considerable attention as the approach appears safe and potentially effective.[20] It has also focused attention on the role of the B cell in the pathogenesis of vasculitis. The development of international collaborative study groups, including the French Vasculitis Study Group, European Vasculitis Study Group (EUVAS) and the International

Study Group for Systemic Vasculitis (INSSYS) has been essential to the development of an evidence base for vasculitis treatment and to the evaluation of newer strategies.[2,6]

Highlights in vasculitis treatment 2003–04

WHAT'S IN?

- A common approach to treating Wegener's granulomatosis and microscopic polyangiitis
- Methotrexate for early and 'non-renal' vasculitis
- Switching from cyclophosphamide to azathioprine or methotrexate after remission induction
- Reduction of cyclophosphamide dose for age and renal impairment, and avoidance of leukopenia
- Prophylaxis against infection, gastric ulceration and corticosteroid-induced osteopenia
- Use of the autoantibodies to neutrophil cytoplasmic antigens (ANCA) test to determine risk of relapse
- Tumor necrosis factor blockade

WHAT'S OUT?

- Long-term daily oral cyclophosphamide
- Short-term, 1-year, regimens: prolonged treatment is required to prevent relapse

WHAT'S NEEDED?

- A safer immunosuppressive than cyclophosphamide for remission induction
- Lower corticosteroid doses
- Earlier diagnosis and institution of effective therapy

References

1. Jayne D. Current attitudes to the therapy of vasculitis. *Kidney Blood Press R* 2003;26:231–9.

2. Jayne D, Rasmussen N, Andrassy K et al. A randomized trial of maintenance therapy for vasculitis associated with antineutrophil cytoplasmic autoantibodies. *N Engl J Med* 2003;349:36–44.

3. de Groot K, Adu D, Savage C. The value of pulse cyclophosphamide in ANCA-associated vasculitis: meta-analysis and critical review. *Nephrol Dial Transplant* 2001;16:2018–27.

4. Jayne D. Update on the European Vasculitis Study Group trials. *Curr Opin Rheumatol* 2001;13:48–55.

5. Guillevin L, Lhote F, Gayraud M et al. Prognostic factors in polyarteritis nodosa and Churg-Strauss syndrome. A prospective study in 342 patients. *Medicine (Baltimore)* 1996;75:17–28.

6. Guillevin L, Cohen P, Mahr A et al. Treatment of polyarteritis nodosa and microscopic polyangiitis with poor prognosis factors: a prospective trial comparing glucocorticoids and six or twelve cyclophosphamide pulses in sixty-five patients. *Arthritis Rheum* 2003;49:93–100.

7. Boomsma MM, Stegeman CA, van der Leij MJ et al. Prediction of relapses in Wegener's granulomatosis by measurement of antineutrophil cytoplasmic antibody levels: a prospective study. *Arthritis Rheum* 2000;43:2025–33.

8. Luqmani RA, Exley AR, Kitas GD et al. Disease assessment and management of the vasculitides. *Baillieres Clin Rheumatol* 1997;11:423–46.

9. Booth AD, Almond MK, Burns A et al. Outcome of ANCA-associated renal vasculitis: a 5-year retrospective study. *Am J Kidney Dis* 2003;41:776–84.

10. Gaskin G, Pusey C. Long-term outcome after immunosuppression and plasma exchange for severe vasculitis-associated glomerulonephritis. *J Am Soc Nephrol* 1999;10:101A.

11. Reinhold-Keller E, Fink CO, Herlyn K et al. High rate of renal relapse in 71 patients with Wegener's granulomatosis under maintenance of remission with low-dose methotrexate. *Arthritis Rheum* 2002;47:326–32.

12. Jayne DR, Chapel H, Adu D et al. Intravenous immunoglobulin for ANCA-associated systemic vasculitis with persistent disease activity. *QJM* 2000;93:433–9.

13. Stegeman CA, Cohen Tervaert JW, De Jong PE et al. Trimethoprim-sulfamethoxazole (co-trimoxazole) for the prevention of relapses of Wegener's granulomatosis. Dutch Co-Trimoxazole Wegener Study Group. *N Engl J Med* 1996;335:16–20.

14. Jayne DR, Rasmussen N. Treatment of antineutrophil cytoplasm autoantibody-associated systemic vasculitis: initiatives of the European Community Systemic Vasculitis Clinical Trials Study Group. *Mayo Clin Proc* 1997;72:737–47.

15. Schmitt WH, Hagen E, Neumann I et al. Treatment of refractory Wegener's granulomatosis with anti-thymocyte globulin (ATG): an open study in 15 patients. *Kidney Int*; in press.

16. Lockwood CM. Refractory Wegener's granulomatosis: a model for shorter immunotherapy of autoimmune diseases. *J R Coll Physicians Lond* 1998;32:473–8.

17. Booth AD, Jefferson HJ, Ayliffe W et al. Safety and efficacy of TNF alpha blockade in relapsing vasculitis. *Ann Rheum Dis* 2002;61:559.

18. Stone JH, Uhlfelder ML, Hellmann DB et al. Etanercept combined with conventional treatment in Wegener's granulomatosis: a six-month open-label trial to evaluate safety. *Arthritis Rheum* 2001;44:1149–54.

19. Birck R, Warnatz K, Lorenz HM et al. 15-Deoxyspergualin in patients with refractory ANCA-associated systemic vasculitis: a six-month open-label trial to evaluate safety and efficacy. *J Am Soc Nephrol* 2003; 14:440–7.

20. Specks U, Fervenza FC, McDonald TJ et al. Response of Wegener's granulomatosis to anti-CD20 chimeric monoclonal antibody therapy. *Arthritis Rheum* 2001;44: 2836–40.

The spondyloarthritides

Juergen Braun MD **and Joachim Sieper** MD
Rheumazentrum Ruhrgebiet, Herne, and Free University Berlin, Germany

This review focuses on the spondyloarthritides (SpA) subtypes, ankylosing spondylitis (AS) and reactive arthritis. Psoriatic arthritis is discussed only briefly, as it is the subject of a separate chapter.

Therapy

Therapeutic options for patients suffering from the more severe forms of SpA have been rather limited. Evidence is now accumulating that anti-tumor necrosis factor (anti-TNF) therapy is highly effective in SpA, particularly in AS and psoriatic arthritis.

Recommendations for anti-TNF therapy in AS were developed by a review of published reports in combination with expert opinion, including a Delphi exercise (a formal consensus method), and a consensus meeting of the Assessments in AS (ASAS) Working Group.[1]

Infliximab. In an open observational extension study of a randomized controlled trial, 78% of 65 AS patients continued to receive infliximab after 1 year at a dose of 5 mg/kg every 6 weeks.[2] At week 54, there was 50% improvement in disease activity in 50% of patients (using the Bath AS disease activity index [BASDAI]).

In an Italian study, 16 patients with peripheral active psoriatic arthritis who had been treated for at least 6 months with methotrexate at a stable dose, were given infliximab, 3 mg/kg every 8 weeks.[3] At week 30, 57% of patients satisfied the American College of Rheumatology (ACR) 70% response rate. The improvement in skin lesions was also significant.

All serious and/or treatment-related adverse events were reported in 107 Belgian patients with SpA treated with infliximab for a total of 192 patient-years.[4] Eight severe infections occurred, including two reactivations of tuberculosis and three retropharyngeal abscesses, and six minor infections with clear bacterial focus. One patient developed a spinocellular carcinoma of the skin. Three AS patients developed palmoplantar pustulosis. All patients recovered completely with adequate treatment. No cases of demyelinating disease or lupus-like syndrome were seen. Infliximab treatment had to be stopped in five patients who had severe infections.

The effect of infliximab treatment on antinuclear antibodies (ANAs), anti-double-stranded DNA (anti-dsDNA), antinucleosome, antihistone and anti-extractable nuclear antigen (anti-ENA) antibodies was examined in 62 patients with rheumatoid arthritis (RA) and 35 SpA patients.[5] Initially, 52% of the RA and 18% of the SpA patients were ANA-positive. After about 30 weeks of infliximab treatment, these prevalences rose significantly, and some RA and SpA patients became positive for IgM and IgA anti-dsDNA antibodies. No IgG anti-dsDNA antibodies or lupus symptoms were observed. The development of other antibodies was not significant.

Etanercept, a 75-kDa-receptor fusion protein, was tested in 30 patients with active AS that had not been treated with disease-modifying antirheumatic drugs or corticosteroids.[6] There was at least a 50% regression of disease activity in 57% of these patients at week 6 compared with 6% of the placebo-treated patients. Disease relapses occurred 6 weeks after etanercept was stopped. No severe adverse events such as major infections were observed during the trial.

Cytokines and autoantigens

Infliximab downregulated both interferon (IFN)γ and tumor necrosis factor (TNF)α secreted by T cells in the peripheral blood of AS patients, but it did not induce a change in the cytokines produced by monocytes during the 3-month period of treatment.[7] In contrast, 12 weeks of etanercept treatment induced a significant increase in the number of IFNγ- and TNFα-positive CD4+ and CD8+ T cells on non-specific stimulation.[8] Neutralization of peripheral TNFα did not induce a downregulation of the ability of

T cells to produce TNFα but caused upregulation, possibly because of a counter-regulatory mechanism.

Based on their human leukocyte antigen (HLA) association, both AS and RA seem to be T-cell-driven diseases in which the autoantigens remain to be defined. One possible autoantigen is the G1 domain of aggrecan, the major cartilage proteoglycan. Spondylitis and erosive polyarthritis have been reported in BALB/c mice immunized with this protein. After antigen-specific stimulation with G1, the CD4+ T cells of 30 AS patients (61.7%) and of 12 RA patients (54.5%) secreted significant amounts of IFNγ and TNFα, while in contrast only 10% of the normal controls showed a response.[9] The relevance of this finding to the pathogenesis of AS and RA remains to be established.

Microbes

PCR was used to detect whether bacterial components were present in synovial-tissue samples from 41 patients with advanced RA, 39 patients with osteoarthritis (OA), and a few with other diseases.[10] Bacterial DNA was not detected using either of the PCR primers in the RA and OA groups. However, confirming previous reports, 5 of 15 synovial fluid samples from patients with reactive arthritis gave a positive result on PCR. Using gas chromatography–mass spectrometry analysis, muramic acid was found in the synovial tissue samples from 4 of 35 RA patients and from 2 of 14 OA patients, but it was not found in the synovial tissue from two patients with undifferentiated arthritis nor from three cadavers.

Elevated levels of anti-*Saccharomyces cerevisiae* IgA antibodies, a marker in Crohn's disease, were found in 108 patients with SpA (43 with AS, 20 with undifferentiated SpA [uSpa], 45 with psoriatic arthritis) compared with 45 healthy controls and 56 patients with RA.[11]

In contrast to another study with lymecycline,[12] an analysis performed 4–7 years after treatment of the initial reactive arthritis suggested that a 3-month course of ciprofloxacin in the acute phase may have a beneficial effect on the long-term prognosis for reactive arthritis.[13]

HLA-B27
Chronic synovitis affects about 10% of patients with severe hemophilia in India. In a study of 473 patients with severe hemophilia (33 of whom had chronic synovitis) and 1175 healthy controls, 64% (21 of 33) of the patients with hemophilia and chronic synovitis were positive for HLA-B27, compared with 5% of those with severe hemophilia but no chronic synovitis (odds ratio 31.6) and 9% of healthy controls.[14] This indicates a strong association between HLA-B27 and chronic synovitis in Indian patients with severe hemophilia.

Synovial membrane
Vascular endothelial growth factor (VEGF) plays a crucial role in angiogenesis. In a study involving 105 patients with SpA, 50 patients with RA and 64 healthy controls, serum VEGF levels were significantly higher among the SpA and RA patients than among the controls.[15] In the SpA patients, serum VEGF levels correlated with disease activity indices, but not with the presence of extra-articular manifestations or syndesmophytes, or with the grade of sacroiliitis.

Imaging
An MRI scoring system was evaluated for assessing spinal inflammation in patients with AS who participated in a randomized placebo-controlled trial of infliximab.[16] The active lesion score, as determined by gadolinium-DTPA, improved by 40% in the infliximab group compared with 6% in the placebo group; the active lesion score as determined by short tau inversion recovery (STIR) sequence improved by 60% in the infliximab group, but deteriorated by 21% in the placebo group. The acute MRI changes correlated with clinical improvement as assessed by the BASDAI.

MRI was performed in 93 patients with SpA and inflammatory back pain for whom radiographs of the sacroiliac joints were available (31 patients with AS and 48 with uSpA).[17] MRI revealed that sacroiliitis was more often bilateral in AS (84%) than in uSpA (48%). Inflammatory changes were found in similar frequency in early and late disease. Involvement of the iliac side was more frequent in early disease. The dorsocaudal parts of the synovial joint and the bone marrow were the most commonly inflamed structures in early disease. In contrast, involvement of the entheses was more common in advanced disease (43% in those with early disease compared with 86% in those with late disease). The HLA-B27-positive patients had more entheseal involvement than the 13 HLA-B27-negative patients. When all pathological changes were assessed, the STIR sequence was less sensitive than the contrast-enhanced sequences – it did not show all relevant changes in 27% of the cases. In particular, inflammation of the cavum was not detected in 15 patients.

Genes

ANKH. The *ANKH* gene is a human homolog of the gene mutated in the murine progressive ankylosis model. In a UK study, sequence variants were identified by genomic sequencing of the 12 *ANKH* exons and their flanking splice sites in 48 AS patients; variants were then screened in 233 patients and 478 controls.[18] Linkage to the *ANKH* locus was assessed in 185 affected-sibling-pair families. Five single-nucleotide polymorphisms (SNPs) were identified within the coding region and flanking splice sites. No association was seen between either susceptibility to AS or its clinical manifestations and these novel polymorphisms, or between disease susceptibility and three known promoter variants. In contrast to another recent study,[19] no linkage was found between the *ANKH* locus and AS.

Vitamin D receptor gene. Osteoporosis is a common finding in AS, and it may contribute to spinal deformity and bone pain. Bone metabolism and inflammatory processes are influenced by the vitamin D receptor gene. On the basis of a recent study from Austria,[20] this gene may account for differences in bone mineral density, in bone metabolism and in inflammatory processes in AS.

NOD2. Chronic inflammatory bowel diseases such as Crohn's disease and ulcerative colitis are disorders interrelated with SpA. The *NOD2* gene has been shown to confer susceptibility to Crohn's disease. In DNA samples from 112 patients with AS and 168 controls with homogeneous Spanish ancestry, there was no evidence that the three most common *NOD2* mutations contribute to AS susceptibility.[21] Therefore, these do not explain the susceptibility locus for AS in chromosome 16q.

CARD15. An insertion mutation at nucleotide 3020 (3020insC) and a missense mutation G2722C in the *CARD15* gene on chromosome 16p have been reported to be associated with Crohn's disease. The protein encoded by the *CARD15* gene is expressed in peripheral monocytes, and regulates apoptosis and NF-κB activation, factors which play an important role in inflammation. In DNA samples from 113 unrelated AS patients and 152 unrelated healthy controls, no significant differences were found between patients and controls in the prevalence of the 3020insC mutation and the G2722C missense mutation.[22]

There is currently no evidence that genes that are probably involved in the pathogenesis of Crohn's disease are also involved in AS. It is not known whether this will change if studies are limited to patients with established Crohn's-disease-like gut lesions.

IL-1B and IL-1RN. Ulcerative colitis and Crohn's disease have been found to be variably associated with the *interleukin (IL)-1B* and *IL-1RN* genes encoding IL-1β and the IL-1-receptor antagonist (IL-1ra). SNPs in the 3' region of the *IL1RN* gene were investigated in a case–control cohort of 394 AS cases and 500 controls.[23] The frequency of allele C at SNP position 30735 in exon 6 was significantly increased in AS (35.1%) compared with controls (27.8%), as was the phenotype frequency (61.7% compared with 48.6%). Taken together, these findings indicate that the *IL-1RN* gene may be associated with AS. In the absence of non-synonymous coding-sequence substitutions, it is possible that the primary disease-associated locus regulates gene expression. Association with specific haplotypes, however, raises the possibility that the primary disease locus is in linkage disequilibrium with a specific combination(s) of markers in the *IL1RN* gene. In this case, the association highlighted could be with a closely linked gene.

IL-10. In a Finnish study, no association with susceptibility to and clinical manifestations of AS was found when three SNPs and two microsatellites lying within the promoter region of the gene encoding IL-10 were studied.[24]

TGFB1. Five intragenic SNPs and three microsatellite markers flanking the *TGFB1* locus were genotyped in 762 individuals from 184 multiplex families.[25] A weak association was noted between the rare *TGFB1* +1632 T allele and AS. The polymorphisms within the *TGFB1* gene play, at most, a small role in AS, implying that other genes encoded on chromosome 19 are involved in AS susceptibility.

A whole-genome linkage scan was performed in 188 affected-sibling-pair families with 454 affected individuals.[26] Heritabilities of the traits were as follows: BASDAI 0.49, Bath AS functional index (BASFI) 0.76, and age at symptom onset 0.33 ($p = 0.005$). No linkage was observed between the major histocompatibility complex (MHC) and any of the traits studied. Significant linkage (logarithm of the odds ratio [LOD] score 4.0) was observed between a region on chromosome 18p and the BASDAI. Age at symptom onset showed linkage to chromosome 11p (LOD score 3.3). Maximum linkage with the BASFI was seen at chromosome 2q (LOD score 2.9). In contrast to the genetic determinants of AS susceptibility, clinical manifestations of the disease measured by the BASDAI, BASFI, and age at symptom onset were largely determined by a small number of genes not encoded within the MHC.[26]

HLA-B27 subtypes. It is known that the HLA-B27 subtypes HLA-B*2706 and HLA-B*2709 are not associated with AS. Since they differ from the strongly associated subtype B*2705 by only one amino acid, this is a striking phenomenon. An analysis of DNA samples from 47 HLA-B27-positive patients with AS and

Highlights in the spondyloarthritides 2003–04

WHAT'S IN?

- Treatment using tumor necrosis factor α blockade
- More sensitive imaging using magnetic resonance
- The concept that genes outside the major histocompatibility complex control clinical manifestations of ankylosing spondylitis

WHAT'S OUT?

- Non-steroidal agents as the only therapy for very active spondylitis

76 HLA-B27-positive healthy controls (19 positive and 57 negative for B*2709) living in different areas of Sardinia revealed that the B27 alleles conferring susceptibility to AS more frequently carried the haplotype (A2;B27;Cw2;DR16) that reaches its highest frequency in patients with AS,[27] while conversely, the non-AS-associated *B*2709* allele is more frequently found together with other HLA alleles that have frequencies inversely correlated with the disease (A32 or A30, Cw1, and DR12). Familial analysis of six individuals positive for HLA-B*2709 confirmed the existence of a 'Sardinian' haplotype that is not associated with AS (A32;B*2709;Cw1;DR12). The authors conclude that in Sardinia, two distinct haplotypes harbor the non-AS-associated *HLA-B*2709* allele and the AS-associated *B27* alleles. These findings are compatible with the hypothesis that genes within the HLA region but other than *HLA-B27* may play some role in conferring susceptibility to AS. In view of other findings, this study argues in favor of a more complex genetic association of AS which involves the HLA class II genes.

References

1. Braun J, Pham T, Sieper J et al. International ASAS consensus statement for the use of anti-tumour necrosis factor agents in patients with ankylosing spondylitis. *Ann Rheum Dis* 2003;62:817–24.

2. Braun J, Brandt J, Listing J et al. Long-term efficacy and safety of infliximab in the treatment of ankylosing spondylitis: an open, observational, extension study of a three-month, randomized, placebo-controlled trial. *Arthritis Rheum* 2003;48:2224–33.

3. Salvarani C, Cantini F, Olivieri I et al. Efficacy of infliximab in resistant psoriatic arthritis. *Arthritis Rheum* 2003;49:541–5.

4. Baeten D, Kruithof E, Van den Bosch F et al. Systematic safety follow up in a cohort of 107 patients with spondyloarthropathy treated with infliximab: a new perspective on the role of host defence in the pathogenesis of the disease? *Ann Rheum Dis* 2003;62:829–34.

5. De Rycke L, Kruithof E, Van Damme N et al. Antinuclear antibodies following infliximab treatment in patients with rheumatoid arthritis or spondylarthropathy. *Arthritis Rheum* 2003;48:1015–23.

6. Brandt J, Khariouzov A, Listing J et al. Six-month results of a double-blind, placebo-controlled trial of etanercept treatment in patients with active ankylosing spondylitis. *Arthritis Rheum* 2003;48:1667–75.

7. Zou J, Rudwaleit M, Brandt J et al. Down-regulation of the non-specific and antigen-specific T cell cytokine response in ankylosing spondylitis during treatment with infliximab. *Arthritis Rheum* 2003;48:780–90.

8. Zou J, Rudwaleit M, Brandt J et al. Up regulation of the production of tumour necrosis factor alpha and interferon gamma by T cells in ankylosing spondylitis during treatment with etanercept. *Ann Rheum Dis* 2003;62:561–4.

9. Zou J, Zhang Y, Thiel A et al. Predominant cellular immune response to the cartilage autoantigenic G1 aggrecan in ankylosing spondylitis and rheumatoid arthritis. *Rheumatology (Oxford)* 2003;42:846–55.

10. Chen T, Rimpilainen M, Luukkainen R et al. Bacterial components in the synovial tissue of patients with advanced rheumatoid arthritis or osteoarthritis: analysis with gas chromatography-mass spectrometry and pan-bacterial polymerase chain reaction. *Arthritis Rheum* 2003;49:328–34.

11. Hoffman IE, Demetter P, Peeters M et al. Anti-saccharomyces cerevisiae IgA antibodies are raised in ankylosing spondylitis and undifferentiated spondyloarthropathy. *Ann Rheum Dis* 2003;62:455–9.

12. Laasila K, Laasonen L, Leirisalo-Repo M. Antibiotic treatment and long term prognosis of reactive arthritis. *Ann Rheum Dis* 2003;62:655–8.

13. Yli-Kerttula T, Luukkainen R, Yli-Kerttula U et al. Effect of a three month course of ciprofloxacin on the late prognosis of reactive arthritis. *Ann Rheum Dis* 2003; 62:880–4.

14. Ghosh K, Shankarkumar U, Shetty S et al. Chronic synovitis and HLA B27 in patients with severe haemophilia. *Lancet* 2003;361: 933–4.

15. Drouart M, Saas P, Billot M et al. High serum vascular endothelial growth factor correlates with disease activity of spondylarthropathies. *Clin Exp Immunol* 2003;132:158–62.

16. Braun J, Baraliakos X, Golder W et al. Magnetic resonance imaging examinations of the spine in patients with ankylosing spondylitis, before and after successful therapy with infliximab: evaluation of a new scoring system. *Arthritis Rheum* 2003;48:1126–36.

17. Muche B, Bollow M, Francois RJ et al. Anatomic structures involved in early- and late-stage sacroiliitis in spondylarthritis: a detailed analysis by contrast-enhanced magnetic resonance imaging. *Arthritis Rheum* 2003;48:1374–84.

18. Timms AE, Zhang Y, Bradbury L et al. Investigation of the role of ANKH in ankylosing spondylitis. *Arthritis Rheum* 2003;48:2898–902.

19. Tsui FW, Tsui HW, Cheng EY et al. Novel genetic markers in the 5'-flanking region of ANKH are associated with ankylosing spondylitis. *Arthritis Rheum* 2003;48:791–7.

20. Obermayer-Pietsch BM, Lange U, Tauber G et al. Vitamin D receptor initiation codon polymorphism, bone density and inflammatory activity of patients with ankylosing spondylitis. *Osteoporos Int* 2003;14:995–1000.

21. Ferreiros-Vidal I, Amarelo J, Barros F et al. Lack of association of ankylosing spondylitis with the most common NOD2 susceptibility alleles to Crohn's disease. *J Rheumatol* 2003;30:102–4.

22. van der Paardt M, Crusius JB, de Koning MH et al. CARD15 gene mutations are not associated with ankylosing spondylitis. *Genes Immun* 2003;4:77–8.

23. Maksymowych WP, Reeve JP, Reveille JD et al. High-throughput single-nucleotide polymorphism analysis of the IL1RN locus in patients with ankylosing spondylitis by matrix-assisted laser desorption ionization-time-of-flight mass spectrometry. *Arthritis Rheum* 2003;48:2011–18.

24. Goedecke V, Crane AM, Jaakkola E et al. Interleukin 10 polymorphisms in ankylosing spondylitis. *Genes Immun* 2003;4:74–6.

25. Jaakkola E, Crane AM, Laiho K et al. The effect of transforming growth factor β1 gene polymorphisms in ankylosing spondylitis. *Rheumatology (Oxford)* 2004;43:32–8.

26. Brown MA, Brophy S, Bradbury L et al. Identification of major loci controlling clinical manifestations of ankylosing spondylitis. *Arthritis Rheum* 2003;48:2234–9.

27. Fiorillo MT, Cauli A, Carcassi C et al. Two distinctive HLA haplotypes harbor the B27 alleles negatively or positively associated with ankylosing spondylitis in Sardinia: implications for disease pathogenesis. *Arthritis Rheum* 2003;48:1385–9.

Psoriatic arthritis

Adrian N Gibbs MB MRCPI and **Douglas J Veale** MD FRCPI FRCP
Department of Rheumatology, St Vincents University Hospital, Dublin, Ireland

Psoriatic arthritis (PsA) is a chronic inflammatory arthritis associated with skin psoriasis in the absence of rheumatoid factor. While initially considered a variant of rheumatoid arthritis (RA), it has emerged as a distinct clinical entity with three main subtypes – polyarticular, oligoarticular and spinal disease.[1] Subsequent studies have revealed that PsA shares a number of genetic, pathogenetic and clinical features with the spondyloarthritides. This concept is supported by magnetic resonance imaging (MRI) studies demonstrating widespread enthesitis in the spondyloarthritides, including PsA, but not in RA.[2]

PsA affects women and men equally, with an incidence of 6/100 000 and a prevalence of about 100/100 000. It occurs in 4–6% of patients with psoriasis and was, until recently, considered to be a relatively benign disease.[3] However, several studies have shown both peripheral and axial disease to be progressive in a significant proportion of patients, reinforcing the need for effective monitoring and treatment.[4–6]

Pathogenesis

The pathogenetic connection between psoriasis and arthritis is not yet clear, though our understanding of the mechanisms of disease has progressed significantly. Numerous factors are key, including immunogenetics, infection, trauma, and changes (e.g. angiogenesis) in the vascular system.[7,8] A number of new candidate genes have been identified, along with novel proinflammatory proteins in the joints. Human leukocyte antigen (HLA) has been implicated as a candidate genetic locus for PsA, with excessive haplotype sharing among affected sibling pairs of individuals with PsA compared with controls.[9] The interleukin (IL)-1 gene complex may play a role in the development of PsA and/or psoriasis, or act as a marker for other genes in the region 2q12 to 2q13.[10] Tumor necrosis factor (TNF)α may also play a role in the development of PsA and/or psoriasis, or a haplotype may act as a marker for other genes on chromosome 6p21.[11] Additionally, TNF gene polymorphisms may be useful prognostic markers in PsA,[12] and a recent study has suggested that bone resorption is mirrored by high numbers of circulating osteoclast precursors.[13] These appear to be derived from TNFα-activated peripheral blood mononuclear cells, which are subsequently exposed to unopposed receptor activator of NF-κB ligand (RANKL) and TNFα in the synovium and subchondral bone (see also Goldring, page 15). *CARD15* represents a pleiotropic autoimmune gene and is the first non-major histocompatibility complex (MHC) gene to be associated with PsA.[14] Local expression of the proinflammatory protein S100A12 (EN-RAGE) in inflamed tissue and its high concentrations in serum suggest a role in PsA, and potential utility as a serum marker.[15]

Imaging
Improved technology for high-resolution ultrasound (HRUS) and MRI has revolutionized diagnosis and assessment of PsA. For example, HRUS has been shown to be highly sensitive in detecting synovitis and tenosynovitis in patients with PsA, particularly in those with associated dactylitis.[16–18]

MRI is particularly sensitive for detecting articular, periarticular and soft tissue inflammation in the peripheral joints and in the spine.[19,20] On fat-suppressed images, diffuse bone edema or osteitis is seen at all sites of entheseal involvement in the spondyloarthritides, which is distinct from RA. Such imaging should permit more appropriately targeted therapy for PsA.

Treatment
Mild arthritis can usually be controlled by anti-inflammatory medication. Because non-steroidal anti-inflammatory agents and cyclooxygenase (Cox)-2-specific drugs can potentially shunt the products of arachidonic acid conversion from the cyclooxygenase to

the lipoxygenase pathway, it has been suggested that the increased leukotriene load might worsen psoriatic skin lesions.[21] However, a recent randomized controlled trial using nimesulide showed no worsening of cutaneous psoriasis.[22]

Systemic glucocorticoids are not advised for protracted use in PsA. The well-known side effects of osteoporosis, infection and glucose intolerance may occur. These drugs may also reduce the efficacy of other disease-modifying antirheumatic drugs (DMARDs) and, on cessation, may lead to rebound worsening of psoriasis.

DMARDs should be instituted early in the course of PsA, particularly if the presentation is polyarticular. The most commonly used agents are methotrexate, sulfasalazine, and ciclosporin. Methotrexate is the DMARD of first choice because of its efficacy in both skin and joint disease; it can also be used with other DMARDs, including ciclosporin,[18] and newer biologics.[23] In a recent randomized controlled trial involving patients with active PsA receiving methotrexate, adding ciclosporin resulted in significant improvements in swollen joint count, C-reactive protein (CRP) and synovitis on HRUS.[18] This suggests combination therapy to be effective in severe disease.

Leflunomide is another anti-inflammatory immunosuppressive agent that has recently been shown to decrease joint count and skin involvement significantly in patients with PsA and psoriasis.[24]

The recognition that a subset of PsA patients respond inadequately to conventional DMARDs, and the doubt relating to the ability of existing DMARDs to prevent joint damage and control spondylitis have led to the use of biological agents. Studies have identified the presence of TNFα in psoriatic skin lesions and inflamed joints,[8,11,25] and anti-TNF therapy has shown promise in controlling peripheral joint synovitis, spondylitis and skin psoriasis.[25–27] The most commonly used anti-TNF drugs at present are infliximab, a chimeric murine–human IgG_1 antibody, and etanercept, a dimeric fusion protein consisting of the extracellular domain of the human p75 TNF receptor linked to the Fc portion of human IgG_1.

Etanercept was well tolerated and provided clinically significant benefit to PsA patients with psoriasis in a double-blind, placebo-

Highlights in **psoriatic arthritis** 2003–04

WHAT'S IN?
- Early intervention
- Aggressive treatment
- Biological targeted therapy
- Imaging – high-resolution ultrasound, magnetic resonance imaging

WHAT'S OUT?
- Psoriatic arthritis as a benign disease
- Prolonged glucocorticoids

WHAT'S NEEDED?
- Agreed diagnostic criteria
- Better predictors of disease progression and treatment response
- Randomized controlled trials of conventional and newer biological agents
- Better understanding of the underlying pathogenesis

controlled trial in 205 patients over 24 weeks, and this was sustained in 169 patients in an open-label extension study.[26]

A small open-label study using infliximab in 16 patients with refractory PsA showed significant improvement in swollen and tender joint counts, pain (measured on a visual-analog scale), patient and physician global assessment, health-assessment questionnaire (HAQ) results and CRP.[23] Infliximab also produced a reduction in cell infiltrate and angiogenic growth factors – vascular endothelial growth factor and angiopoietin 2 – that paralleled a dramatic clinical response in skin and joints.[25] Other biological therapies proposed for use in PsA aim to interfere with T cells, which are present in the inflammatory infiltrate found in skin lesions and synovium. A recent study using the non-Fc-receptor-binding humanized derivative of a murine anti-CD3 antibody demonstrated considerable improvement of synovitis within 1 month in six of seven patients in an open-label study.[28] Alefacept, a leukocyte-function-associated-3 (LFA-3)-IgG$_1$ fusion protein, was also shown to improve both skin disease and synovitis in an open-label trial.[29]

References

1. Veale D, Rogers S, FitzGerald O. Classification of clinical subsets in psoriatic arthritis. *Br J Rheumatol* 1994;33:133–8.

2. McGonagle D, Gibbon W, O'Connor P et al. Characteristic magnetic resonance imaging entheseal changes of knee synovitis in spondyloarthropathy. *Arthritis Rheum* 1998;41:694–799.

3. Shbeeb M, Uramoto KM, Gibson LE et al. The epidemiology of psoriatic arthritis in Olmsted County, Minnesota, USA, 1982-91. *J Rheumatol* 2000;27:1247–50.

4. Veale DJ. The epidemiology of psoriatic arthritis: fact or fiction? *J Rheumatol* 2000; 27:1105–7.

5. Kane D, Stafford L, Bresnihan B et al. A prospective, clinical and radiological study of early psoriatic arthritis: an early synovitis clinic experience. *Rheumatology (Oxford)* 2003;42:1460–8.

6. McHugh NJ, Balachrishnan C, Jones SM. Progression of peripheral joint disease in psoriatic arthritis: a 5-yr prospective study. *Rheumatology* 2003;42:778–83.

7. Fearon U, Veale DJ. Pathogenesis of psoriatic arthritis (review). *Clin Exp Dermatol* 2001;26:333–7.

8. Fearon U, Griosios K, Fraser A et al. Angiopoietins, growth factors, and vascular morphology in early arthritis. *J Rheumatol* 2003;30: 260–8.

9. Gladman DD, Farewell VT, Pellett F et al. HLA is a candidate region for psoriatic arthritis. Evidence for excessive HLA sharing in sibling pairs. *Hum Immunol* 2003;64:887–9.

10. Ravindran JS, Owen P, Lagan P et al. Interleukin 1 α, interleukin 1 β and interleukin 1 receptor gene polymorphisms in psoriatic arthritis. *Rheumatology (Oxford)* 2004;43:22–6.

11. Ravindran JS, Lagan A, Ahmad T et al. TNF alpha haplotypes are associated with psoriatic arthritis. *Arthritis Rheum* 2003;48:S411.

12. Balding J, Kane D, Livingstone W et al. Cytokine gene polymorphisms: association with psoriatic arthritis susceptibility and severity. *Arthritis Rheum* 2003;48:1408–13.

13. Ritchlin CT, Haas-Smith SA, Li P et al. Mechanisms of TNF-alpha- and RANKL-mediated osteoclastogenesis and bone resorption in psoriatic arthritis. *J Clin Invest* 2003;111:821–31.

14. Rahman P, Bartlett S, Siannis F et al. CARD15: a pleiotropic autoimmune gene that confers susceptibility to psoriatic arthritis. *Am J Hum Genet* 2003;73:677–81.

15. Foell D, Kane D, Bresnihan B et al. Expression of the pro-inflammatory protein S100A12 (EN-RAGE) in rheumatoid and psoriatic arthritis. *Arthritis Rheum* 2003;48:1408–13.

16. Kane D, Greney T, Bresnihan B et al. Ultrasonography in the diagnosis and management of psoriatic dactylitis. *J Rheumatol* 1999;26:1746–51.

17. Wakefield RJ, Emery P, Veale DJ. Ultrasonography and psoriatic arthritis. *J Rheumatol* 2000;27:1564–5.

18. Fraser AD, van Kuryk A, Westhovens R et al. A randomised, double-blind, placebo controlled multi-centre trial of combination therapy with methotrexate plus cyclosporin vs methotrexate plus placebo in patients with active psoriatic arthritis (PsA). *Arthritis Rheum* 2003;48:S170.

19. Offidani A, Collini I, Valeri G et al. Subclinical joint involvement in psoriasis: magnetic resonance imaging and X-ray findings. *Acta Derm Venereol* 1998;78:463–5.

20. Marzo-Ortega H, McGonagle DM, O'Connor P et al. Efficacy of etanercept in the treatment of the entheseal pathology in resistant spondyloarthropathy: a clinical and magnetic resonance imaging study. *Arthritis Rheum* 2001;44:2112–17.

21. Griffiths CE. Therapy for psoriatic arthritis: sometimes a conflict for psoriasis. *Br J Rheumatol* 1997;36:409–10.

22. Sarzi-Puttini P, Santandrea S, Boccassini L et al. The role of NSAIDs in psoriatic arthritis: evidence from a controlled study with nimesulide. *Clin Exp Rheumatol* 2001;19:S17–20.

23. Salvarani C, Cantini F, Olivieri I et al. Efficacy of infliximab in resistant psoriatic arthritis. *Arthritis Rheum* 2003;49:541–5.

24. Mease P, Nash P, Gladman DD et al. Leflunomide in the treatment of psoriatic arthritis: joint and skin efficacy and safety in the TOPAS study. *Arthritis Rheum* 2003; 48:S169.

25. Veale DJ, Markham T, Fearon U et al. Therapy in psoriasis and psoriatic arthritis: anti-TNFα clinical and angiogenic responses. *Arthritis Rheum* 2003;49:S168.

26. Mease P, Ruderman E, Kivitz A et al. Continued efficacy of etanercept (Enbrel) in patients with psoriatic arthritis and psoriasis. *Arthritis Rheum* 2003;48:S169.

27. Marzo-Ortega H, McGonagle D, Veale D et al. Case definition of psoriatic arthritis. *Lancet* 2000;356:2095 (discussion 2096).

28. Utset TO, Auger JA, Peace D et al. Modified anti-CD3 therapy in psoriatic arthritis: a phase I/II clinical trial. *J Rheumatol* 2002;29: 1907–13.

29. Kraan MC, van Kuijk AW, Dinant HJ et al. Alefacept treatment in psoriatic arthritis: reduction of the effector T cell population in peripheral blood and synovial tissue is associated with improvement of clinical signs of arthritis. *Arthritis Rheum* 2002;46:2776–84.

Juvenile idiopathic arthritis

Kiran Nistala BA MSc MRCP **and Tauny Southwood** BM BS FRACP FRCPA FRCP FRCPCH

Department of Paediatric Rheumatology, Birmingham Children's Hospital, and Institute of Child Health, University of Birmingham, UK

There have been recent advances in the understanding and treatment of many chronic inflammatory diseases in humans, including juvenile idiopathic arthritis (JIA). There is an urgent need for further research, however. In a cohort study with a mean follow-up period of 10 years, fewer than half the children affected by JIA had achieved disease remission (no signs of disease activity in the absence of antirheumatic therapy for at least 6 months) at the last visit.1 Furthermore, for those affected by JIA, unemployment in adulthood is three times the national average.[2]

Knowledge extrapolated from research into adults with chronic inflammatory diseases, such as rheumatoid arthritis (RA), must be interpreted with caution, as important differences exist between arthritides in children and in adults. JIA appears to be a more heterogeneous disease than RA, with a number of clinically distinct subtypes, of which the most common is oligoarthritis (Table 1).[3] The complications of JIA further emphasize important differences from RA, including local and generalized growth disturbances, delayed maturation and asymptomatic chronic anterior uveitis. Immunogenetic differences are also notable. Human leukocyte antigen (HLA)-DR4, a prominent genetic association with RA, is not associated with most forms of JIA. Rheumatoid factor is found in fewer than 5% of patients with JIA, suggesting B-cell abnormalities have less of a role in the majority of JIA cases. The central pathology for both RA and JIA, however, is remarkably similar – inflamed synovium.

TABLE 1
Classification of juvenile idiopathic arthritis (International League Against Rheumatism/WHO)

Juvenile idiopathic arthritis (JIA): arthritis of unknown etiology, beginning before the 16th birthday and persisting for at least 6 weeks, excluding other known conditions. NB all categories of JIA are non-overlapping*

Systemic:	Arthritis in one or more joints, with or preceded by daily fever for at least 2 weeks (documented to be quotidian for at least 3 days), accompanied by at least **one** of: <ul><li>evanescent (non-fixed) erythematous rash</li><li>generalized lymph node enlargement</li><li>hepatomegaly and/or splenomegaly</li><li>serositis</li></ul>
Polyarticular:	Arthritis affecting more than four joints in the first 6 months of disease
RF negative:	A test for rheumatoid factor (RF) is negative
RF positive:	Two or more tests for RF (at least 3 months apart during the first 6 months of disease) are positive
Oligoarticular:	Arthritis affecting one to four joints during the first 6 months of disease
Persistent:	Arthritis affecting no more than four joints throughout the disease course
Extended:	Arthritis affecting a total of more than four joints after the first 6 months of disease
Enthesitis-related arthritis:	Arthritis and enthesitis or arthritis or enthesitis and at least **two** of: <ul><li>sacroiliac joint tenderness/inflammatory lumbosacral pain</li><li>HLA B27</li><li>acute anterior uveitis</li><li>onset of arthritis in boys > 6 years old</li><li>family history of HLA B27-associated disease</li></ul>

(CONTINUED)

TABLE 1 (CONTINUED)

Psoriatic arthritis:	Arthritis and psoriasis or arthritis and at least **two** of: • dactylitis • nail pitting or onycholysis • first-degree relative with psoriasis

*JIA fulfilling criteria for more than one category, or JIA not fulfilling criteria for any category, is regarded as undifferentiated JIA

Histopathology

Microscopic evaluation of inflamed synovium shows marked hyperplasia due to an accumulation of macrophages and fibroblast-like synoviocytes in the lining layer. In the sublining layer, there is infiltration of T cells, plasma cells, mast cells and natural killer (NK) cells. In arthritis, the T-cell aggregate is present very early in the disease and is predominantly made up of $CD4^+$ cells, though some clinical subtype-specific alterations in CD4:8 ratios have been observed in JIA.[4] Degradative enzymes, such as metalloproteinases, are found in the inflammatory infiltrate in association with pannus formation, and cartilage and bone destruction.[5] Interest in the role of regulatory ($CD4^+$, $CD25^+$) T cells in this process is emerging. In JIA, the interleukin (IL)-10-producing $CD4^+$ $CD30^+$ T cell has been associated with disease remission.[6]

Innate immunity and initiation of inflammation

Sibling studies have suggested an important, though incomplete, role for genetic factors in the pathogenesis of JIA. As a result, environmental agents, and in particular infectious agents, have been sought to explain the initiation and perpetuation of JIA. It is well known that infection with enteric bacteria acts as a precipitant for reactive arthritis. Immune responses to bacterial components and molecular evidence of bacterial DNA have been found in the synovial fluid and peripheral blood of those with JIA.[7,8] It is interesting to speculate that the variable expression of Toll-like receptors (TLR), which are cell-surface pattern-recognition molecules, may provide a link between a genetic predisposition to chronic inflammation and environmental exposure to pathogens, as demonstrated in animal models.[9] Preliminary data, however, suggest that TLR4 polymorphisms are not associated with JIA (W Thompson, ARC Epidemiology Research Unit, UK and T Southwood, unpublished observations).

Adaptive immune system

If activation of the innate immune system is the trigger for inflammation, the prominent and early accumulation of T cells in synovium suggests a role for these cells in its perpetuation. The synovial T-cell population is in a dynamic state of flux between factors that promote T-cell recruitment, division, emigration and death.

T-cell recruitment. Recruitment of T cells into the joint requires initial binding to the endothelium before transmigration through the basement membrane. This depends on a family of adhesion molecules (including selectin and intercellular adhesion molecules [ICAMs]) expressed by endothelial cells in response to cytokines such as IL-1 and tumor necrosis factor (TNF)α. In animal models of JIA, upregulation of selectin ligands in T cells increases the accumulation of these cells into synovial tissue, suggesting an important role for chemokines in enhancing T-cell recruitment to the synovium.[10] In JIA synovium, levels of ICAM1 and selectin correlate with measures of disease activity; lower levels predict a better response to intra-articular injection.[11] Other T-cell integrins, such as the site-specific gut-mucosa-associated integrin α4β7 and synovial αFβ7, may be involved in T-cell recruitment in JIA.[12] These findings may have therapeutic significance, as blocking adhesion molecules may minimize T-cell recruitment and halt inflammation at an early stage.

T-cell division. Antigen-specific synovial T cells are likely to be present, but at low frequencies (1:500–1:2000) and dividing T cells account for less than 1% of the synovial T cell population in JIA.[13] It is likely, however, that the T cell has an important role in the pathogenesis of JIA, as evidence of oligoclonality in the intra-articular T-cell population has been demonstrated in JIA, suggesting that the trimolecular complex (recognition of major histocompatibility complex [MHC]–peptide complexes by T-cell receptors) plays a role in the pathogenesis of juvenile arthritis.[14]

T-cell retention. The stimulus to retain T cells within the inflamed joint in JIA is unclear. Chemokines regulate the migration of leukocytes between tissue compartments via specific receptors. Elevated synovial levels of the chemokine stromal cell-derived factor (SDF)-1 and its receptor CXCR4 have been found in RA.[15] The inducible chemokine receptors CXCR3, a cell-surface receptor for the proinflammatory chemokines IP-10 and Mig, and CCR5, which binds macrophage inflammatory protein 1α and 1β, RANTES, and members of the monocyte chemotactic protein family, are upregulated on infiltrating T cells in JIA.[12,16] It is likely that expression of the inducible chemokine receptors favors synovial T-cell accumulation and retention in JIA joints.

T-cell death. During normal recovery from tissue inflammation, programmed cell death (apoptosis) contributes to the resolution of the inflammatory cellular infiltrate while minimizing bystander cell damage. Apoptosis via the Fas signaling pathway has been shown to be upregulated in JIA, but this may be an epiphenomenon of a high inflammatory state.[17,18] T cells from synovial fluid may survive despite expressing CD95, a marker for Fas-mediated apoptosis.[18] Apoptosis has also been shown to be disrupted in RA because type-1 interferons (IFNs) prolong T-cell survival,[19] but this mechanism has yet to be demonstrated in JIA.

A further insight into defective apoptosis has come from studying patients with systemic arthritis, particularly those with a hemophagocytic complication known as macrophage-activation syndrome. NK cells normally play a homeostatic role in inducing apoptosis through perforin/granzyme B-mediated cell-wall puncture.

NK cells from these patients have lower activity and produce reduced levels of perforin.[20] Activated T cells are no longer controlled by apoptosis and, instead, produce high levels of TNF and IFNγ that may lead to macrophage activation. Autologous hemopoietic stem-cell transplantation has been shown to correct the perforin defect.[21]

Cytokine imbalance and T cells

There is convincing evidence that factors controlling T-cell dynamics are disordered in arthritis. Is there a common etiology underlying the demonstrated abnormalities of adhesion molecules, chemokines and apoptosis? All three are influenced by the cytokine microenvironment in the joint either indirectly, by acting on endothelial cells and macrophages, or directly in the case of apoptosis. Factors that account for disturbed cytokine production could explain the abnormal persistence of T cells that occurs in JIA. One such explanation may be found in recent evidence linking specific cytokine polymorphisms to JIA.[22,23] In this model, the risk of developing JIA and its severity depend on the levels of TNF (proinflammatory) and IL-10 (anti-inflammatory) cytokines produced. It is important to note that such polymorphisms may be JIA-subtype specific. For example, IL-6 abnormalities appear to be associated with systemic arthritis only.[24]

T cells secrete as well as respond to cytokines and there is good evidence for a predominantly T helper (T_{h1}) or proinflammatory pattern of secretion in JIA.[25] Intriguingly, the switch from T_{h1} to T_{h2} could account for the higher remission rates of oligoarthritis relative to those of polyarthritis and RA.[26]

Moving on – the role of the fibroblast

T cells have been the focus of research into JIA for some time, but recent evidence from RA is challenging their dominance. Buckley et al. have shown that fibroblasts from patients with RA produce T-cell-recruiting, pro-survival (IFNβ) and retentive (SDF-1) factors and may even be involved in T_h-class switching.[27] Studies of fibroblasts in JIA are beginning to emerge that corroborate this picture. Synovial fibroblasts from JIA, but not other arthritides, produce high levels of proinflammatory cytokines and have morphological abnormalities suggestive of deregulated proliferation.[28] The fibroblast-derived stromal microenvironment may favor T-cell retention and persistent inflammation.

Therapeutic advances

Advances in the understanding of the molecular basis of JIA have been accompanied by improvements in clinical research methodology. Examples include a new disease classification (allowing greater clarity in the study of clinically homogeneous disease subgroups), and a set of validated core-outcome variables (COVs), which enable the reproducible measurement of therapeutic responses. These advances have improved our understanding of the variability in therapeutic responses to methotrexate (MTX): children with extended oligoarthritis respond better to MTX than those with systemic arthritis.[29]

Anti-TNF therapy

The investigation of etanercept, a soluble TNFα receptor, and other 'biological' therapies targeting molecules in the pathway of inflammation have widened the therapeutic armamentarium for JIA. Etanercept is the first biological agent to be licensed for use in children. It exerts a functional TNF blockade by binding to TNF with a much greater avidity than naturally occurring TNF receptors. It has been successful at controlling polyarthritis in children. Follow-up data at 2 years show that 80% of polyarthritis patients resistant to MTX had a 50% improvement in COVs.[30]

Another TNF blocker, infliximab, a chimeric human–murine monoclonal antibody against TNFα, has been studied in an open-label prospective European trial. Nine of the original 24 patients with active disease refractory to standard treatment showed a rapid improvement with infliximab infusions and maintained their response at 2 years.[31]

Other recent trials of biologics include a Phase II trial of anti-IL-6

> ### Highlights in juvenile idiopathic arthritis 2003–04
>
> **WHAT'S IN?**
> - A rigorous classification scheme to underpin research in juvenile idiopathic arthritis (JIA)
> - Non-HLA genes in the predisposition to JIA
> - Involvement of fibroblasts, antigen-presenting cells, and natural killer cells in the pathogenesis of JIA
> - 'Disease-specific' disruption in cytokine networks
> - The use of targeted biological therapy to control unremitting joint inflammation
>
> **WHAT'S OUT?**
> - The terms 'Still's disease', 'juvenile rheumatoid arthritis (JRA)' and 'juvenile chronic arthritis' (JCA)
> - The concept that synovial inflammation is due solely to in-situ T-cell proliferation
> - Benign prognosis: "It's only juvenile arthritis; they grow out of it"
> - The use of traditional disease-modifying anti-rheumatic drugs (gold, penicillamine) to control arthritis

receptor antibody (MRA) in children with systemic arthritis,[32] and a pilot investigation of CTLA4-Ig (see also page 101).

Bone marrow transplantation

A small proportion of children with severe polyarticular or systemic arthritis continue to get progressive joint destruction, growth failure and disabling side effects from conventional medication. Autologous stem cell transplant has been carried out in children with severe refractory JIA, with encouraging results: 21 of 25 children maintained remission or had mild relapses only at a median follow-up of 33 months.[33] Initially, there was a significant treatment-related mortality, possibly due to indolent pre-existing infections and subsequent macrophage activation syndrome post transplant; this has now been addressed by careful case selection.

References

1. Fantini F, Gerloni V, Gattinara M et al. Remission in juvenile chronic arthritis: a cohort study of 683 consecutive cases with a mean 10 year followup. *J Rheumatol* 2003;30:579–84.

2. Packham JC, Hall MA. Long-term follow-up of 246 adults with juvenile idiopathic arthritis: education and employment. *Rheumatology (Oxford)* 2002;41:1436–9.

3. Petty RE, Southwood TR, Baum J et al. Revision of the proposed classification criteria for juvenile idiopathic arthritis: Durban 1997. *J Rheumatol* 1998;25:1991–4.

4. Murray KJ, Luyrink L, Grom AA et al. Immunohistological characteristics of T cell infiltrates in different forms of childhood onset chronic arthritis. *J Rheumatol* 1996;23:2116–24.

5. Gattorno M, Gerloni V, Morando A et al. Synovial membrane expression of matrix metalloproteinases and tissue inhibitor 1 in juvenile idiopathic arthritides. *J Rheumatol* 2002; 29:1774–9.

6. de Kleer IM, Kamphuis SM, Rijkers GT et al. The spontaneous remission of juvenile idiopathic arthritis is characterized by CD30+ T cells directed to human heat-shock protein 60 capable of producing the regulatory cytokine interleukin-10. *Arthritis Rheum* 2003;48:2001–10.

7. Pacheco-Tena C, Alvarado De La Barrera C, Lopez-Vidal Y et al. Bacterial DNA in synovial fluid cells of patients with juvenile onset spondyloarthropathies. *Rheumatology* 2001;40:920–7.

8. Bibi F, Ryder CAJ, Gardner-Medwin JM et al. Molecular detection of bacterial DNA in synovial fluid and peripheral blood of children with juvenile idiopathic arthritis. *Rheumatology* 2002; 41(suppl 1):4.

9. Ronaghy A, Prakken BJ, Takabayashi K et al. Immunostimulatory DNA sequences influence the course of adjuvant arthritis. *J Immunol* 2002;168:51–6.

10. De Benedetti F, Pignatti P, Biffi M et al. Increased expression of alpha(1,3)-fucosyltransferase-VII and P-selectin binding of synovial fluid T cells in juvenile idiopathic arthritis. *J Rheumatol* 2003;30:1611–15.

11. Bloom BJ, Nelson SM, Alario AJ et al. Synovial fluid levels of E-selectin and intercellular adhesion molecule-1: relationship to joint inflammation in children with chronic arthritis. *Rheumatol Int* 2002;22:175–7.

12. Black AP, Bhayani H, Ryder CA et al. An association between the acute phase response and patterns of antigen induced T cell proliferation in juvenile idiopathic arthritis. *Arthritis Res Ther* 2003:R277–84.

13. Black AP, Bhayani H, Ryder CA et al. T-cell activation without proliferation in juvenile idiopathic arthritis. *Arthritis Res* 2002;4: 177–83.

14. Wedderburn LR, Patel A, Varsani H et al. Divergence in the degree of clonal expansions in inflammatory T cell subpopulations mirrors HLA-associated risk alleles in genetically and clinically distinct subtypes of childhood arthritis. *Int Immunol* 2001;13:1541–50.

15. Buckley CD, Amft N, Bradfield PF et al. Persistent induction of the chemokine receptor CXCR4 by TGF-beta 1 on synovial T cells contributes to their accumulation within the rheumatoid synovium. *J Immunol* 2000;165:3423–9.

16. Wedderburn LR, Robinson N, Patel A et al. Selective recruitment of polarized T cells expressing CCR5 and CXCR3 to the inflamed joints of children with juvenile idiopathic arthritis. *Arthritis Rheum* 2000; 43:765–74.

17. Smolewska E, Brozik H, Smolewski P et al. Apoptosis of peripheral blood lymphocytes in patients with juvenile idiopathic arthritis. *Ann Rheum Dis* 2003; 62:761–3.

18. Knipp S, Feyen O, Ndagijimana J et al. Ex vivo apoptosis, CD95 and CD28 expression in T cells of children with juvenile idiopathic arthritis. *Rheumatol Int* 2003; 23:112–15.

19. Akbar AN, Salmon M. Cellular environments and apoptosis: tissue microenvironments control activated T-cell death (review). *Immunol Today* 1997;18:72–6.

20. Grom AA, Villanueva J, Lee S et al. Natural killer cell dysfunction in patients with systemic-onset juvenile rheumatoid arthritis and macrophage activation syndrome. *J Pediatr* 2003; 142:292–6.

21. Wulffraat NM, Rijkers GT, Elst E et al. Reduced perforin expression in systemic juvenile idiopathic arthritis is restored by autologous stem-cell transplantation. *Rheumatology (Oxford)* 2003;42:375–9.

22. Zeggini E, Thomson W, Kwiatkowski D et al. British Paediatric Rheumatology Study Group. Linkage and association studies of single-nucleotide polymorphism-tagged tumor necrosis factor haplotypes in juvenile oligoarthritis. *Arthritis Rheum* 2002;46:3304–11.

23. Crawley E, Kay R, Sillibourne J et al. Polymorphic haplotypes of the interleukin-10 5' flanking region determine variable interleukin-10 transcription and are associated with particular phenotypes of juvenile rheumatoid arthritis. *Arthritis Rheum* 1999;42:1101–8.

24. Pignatti P, Vivarelli M, Meazza C et al. Abnormal regulation of interleukin 6 in systemic juvenile idiopathic arthritis. *J Rheumatol* 2001;28:1670–6.

25. Scola MP, Thompson SD, Brunner HI et al. Interferon-gamma:interleukin 4 ratios and associated type 1 cytokine expression in juvenile rheumatoid arthritis synovial tissue. *J Rheumatol* 2002; 29:369–78.

26. Gattorno M, Prigione I, Chiesa S et al. Flexibility of TH1 cytokine expression with JIA. *Arthritis Rheum* 2003;48(suppl):abstr 139.

27. Buckley CD, Pilling D, Lord JM et al. Fibroblasts regulate the switch from acute resolving to chronic persistent inflammation (review). *Trends Immunol* 2001;22:199–204.

28. Fawcett LB, Fawcett PT, Vinette KMB et al. Culture and characteristics of synovial fibroblast like cells from samples of synovial fluid obtained from patients with JRA. *Arthritis Rheum* 2003; 48(suppl):abstr 151.

29. Woo P, Southwood TR, Prieur AM et al. Randomized, placebo-controlled, crossover trial of low-dose oral methotrexate in children with extended oligoarticular or systemic arthritis. *Arthritis Rheum* 2000; 43:1849–57.

30. Lovell DJ, Giannini EH, Reiff A et al. Long-term efficacy and safety of etanercept in children with polyarticular-course juvenile rheumatoid arthritis: interim results from an ongoing multicenter, open-label, extended-treatment trial. *Arthritis Rheum* 2003;48:218–26.

31. Gerloni V, Pontikaki M, Gattinara A et al. Efficacy effusions of infliximab in persistently active refractory JIA. *Clinical Exp Rheum* 2003;21(suppl):abstr 52.

32. Yokota S, Miyamae T, Imagawa T et al. Phase II trial of anti IL6 receptor antibody (MRA) for children with systemic onset JIA. *Arthritis Rheum* 2003;48(suppl):abstr 1070.

33. Wulffraat NM, Brinkman D, Ferster A et al. Long term follow up of autologous stem cell transplantation for refractory JIA. *Bone Marrow Transplant* 2003;32(suppl 1):S61–4.

Cytokine blockade

Henry Townsend MD **and Larry Moreland** MD
Division of Clinical Immunology and Rheumatology, University of Alabama at Birmingham, USA

Multiple cytokines operate as a network in a redundant and overlapping manner in inflammatory rheumatic diseases (Figure 1).[1–3] This review highlights recent data on tumor necrosis factor (TNF)α and interleukin (IL)-1 inhibitors, as well as new cytokine targets under investigation as therapies for rheumatoid arthritis (RA).

Proinflammatory cytokine targets

TNFα is a multipotent proinflammatory cytokine that plays a critical role in the synovial proliferation, cartilage and bone destruction, and systemic inflammation that characterize RA.[1,3,4] Two anti-TNFα monoclonal antibodies (infliximab and adalimumab) and a soluble TNF receptor–Fc fusion molecule (etanercept) are approved (USA and UK) for the treatment of RA. Despite being the most significant therapeutic development for the treatment of RA in the last two decades, in clinical trials, approximately one-third of patients treated with these agents do not meet American College of Rheumatology (ACR) 20% response criteria. Also noteworthy is a phenomenon of waning efficacy with increasing duration of use in some patients receiving TNFα inhibitors. The biology underlying both these observations remains an area of investigation. Clearly defining why RA patients respond, or do not respond, to various therapies will guide development of future therapeutic strategies for treating RA.

The recently presented ASPIRE and TEMPO trials provide data that combination therapy with anti-TNFα agents and methotrexate has better efficacy (signs and symptoms, and radiographic results) compared with anti-TNFα or methotrexate monotherapy (from

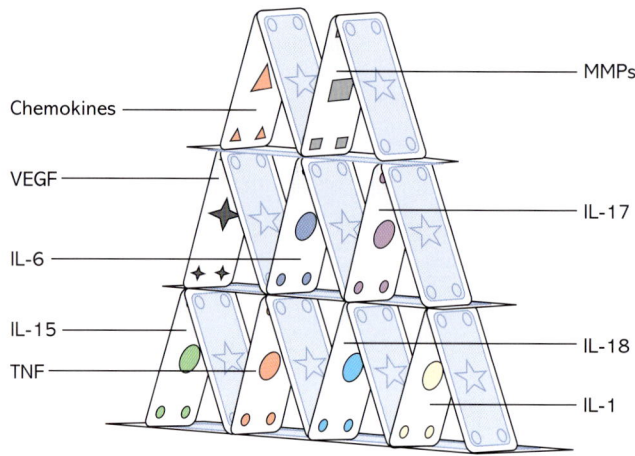

Figure 1 The inflammatory house of cards. The findings that many cytokines are involved in the generation of the inflammatory and destructive events characteristic of rheumatoid arthritis, as well as the significant and similar efficacy of targeting different cytokines in clinical trials, but the rare occurrence of remissions, suggest a multiplicity and redundancy of these events. This is depicted here as a house of cards: pulling one card – that is, interference with one target – breaks part of this 'inflammatory composite'. However, no single card, when eliminated, seems to be sufficient to allow the collapse of the whole inflammatory construct. Rather, it might be necessary to interfere with more than one molecule to fully block the events. MMP, matrix metalloproteinase; VEGF, vascular endothelial growth factor; IL, interleukin; TNF, tumor necrosis factor. Reproduced with permission.[1]

presentations made at the 2003 annual meetings of the European League Against Rheumatism and the ACR, respectively). It remains to be determined if the less expensive triple therapy (methotrexate, sulfasalazine and hydroxychloroquine) combination, or other disease-modifying antirheumatic drug combinations, will provide similar clinical responses to those gained with anti-TNFα plus methotrexate. Such studies are now under way.

Alternative methods of TNFα inhibition are also under development. CNP870, a pegylated Fab fragment of a humanized monoclonal anti-TNFα IgG, has been shown to reduce disease activity in Phase II RA studies.[4] Onercept, a fusion protein of recombinant human TNF receptor-1 (TNF-R1, also known as p55) with IgG_1, is in development for RA. TNFα-converting enzyme (TACE) is a matrix metalloproteinase that cleaves surface-bound TNFα to release soluble cytokine.[5] Because TACE is overexpressed in rheumatoid synovium, it is speculated that inhibiting the release of soluble TNFα may reduce inflammation in patients with high TNFα levels. Orally bioavailable TACE inhibitors have shown efficacy in animal models of inflammatory arthritis and are now in human trials.

Adverse effects of TNFα inhibitors. As with most immunosuppressive therapies, the risk of serious infections is higher in patients using TNFα inhibitors. To date, tuberculosis (TB) has been the infection of most significance. Worldwide, there have been approximately 300 cases of TB in patients taking these drugs. Half of the TB cases have been the more serious disseminated form of TB.[6] Other serious infections reported in patients using anti-TNF therapies include fungal infections, *Pneumocystis carinii*, listeria, and cytomegalovirus infections. The overall rate of serious infections for patients treated with TNF inhibitors is 2–3%.[6]

TNFα inhibitors pose other risks besides increased vulnerability to infections. Post-marketing surveillance has revealed case reports of a demyelinating disease similar to multiple sclerosis in patients taking these drugs.[6] Anti-TNF therapy has also been associated with congestive heart failure – not only exacerbations in patients with known heart failure, but also first episodes of heart failure.[7] Deaths due to heart failure have been reported, prompting the manufacturers of these drugs to issue warnings of this risk to both doctors and patients. Other observed adverse events with these agents include cytopenias, lymphoproliferative disorders, and a lupus-like syndrome. The true causal relationships and prevalence of these events remains an area of investigation.

IL-1 has many similarities to TNFα and it is now well established as another key proinflammatory cytokine involved in RA. Like TNFα, it is overexpressed in rheumatoid synovium, and it exists in a membrane-bound precursor form that requires enzymatic cleavage into the active soluble cytokine.[1] Two different IL-1 receptors exist: type I receptors are present on T cells, endothelial cells and fibroblasts, whereas type II receptors predominate on B cells, monocytes and neutrophils.[1,2]

Anakinra is a recombinant form of IL-1 receptor antagonist (IL-1RA). IL-1RA is a naturally occurring IL-1 receptor ligand that competes with IL-1 for binding to the cell surface IL-1 receptor, but does not induce intracellular signaling when bound.[2] Anakinra is the first IL-1-blocking drug approved for the treatment of RA (USA and UK). Several other IL-1-inhibiting agents are in development. A soluble, recombinant type II IL-1 receptor has shown preclinical efficacy and is currently in early-phase clinical trials in RA. IL-1 Trap is a novel recombinant molecule consisting of IL-1RI and IL-1-receptor accessory protein (IL-1Rac) fused to human IgGFc.[1,2] Phase II trials of this agent in RA patients are in progress. Lastly, IL-1 and another proinflammatory cytokine, IL-18, must be liberated from a precursor form to become an active soluble cytokine. This process is mediated by IL-1-converting enzyme (ICE). Several ICE inhibitors are under development and one agent, pralnacasan, has entered Phase III clinical trials in RA.[1]

IL-6 is a proinflammatory cytokine that is consistently found at high levels in RA synovial fluid. Its numerous proinflammatory effects include stimulation of T-cell proliferation, B-cell and osteoclast differentiation, and leukocyte chemotaxis.[8] A Phase I/II study in which a single intravenous dose of humanized IL-6 receptor (IL-6R) monoclonal antibody was administered to RA patients resulted in normalization of C-reactive protein (CRP).[8] Phase II clinical trials evaluating this same agent are in progress.

IL-15 is present in high concentrations in RA joints, where its many properties include stimulation of T-cell chemotaxis, activation and proliferation.[1] IL-15 blockade in murine and primate models of collagen-induced arthritis, and in a Phase I trial in humans with RA have all showed promising results.[1,2]

IL-18 is a proinflammatory cytokine that, like IL-1, is derived from its precursor by ICE.[9] IL-18 upregulates the production of TNFα, IL-1, and granulocyte-macrophage colony-stimulating factor (GM-CSF) by synovial-lining macrophages. In addition, the combination of IL-18 with IL-12 or IL-15 induces production of interferon (IFN)γ.[9] Current targets for blocking IL-18 activity include ICE inhibitors, anti-IL-18 monoclonal antibody and a recombinant form of IL-18-binding protein (IL-18bp). Administration of anti-IL-18 monoclonal antibody and IL-18bp to mice with collagen-induced arthritis reduced synovial TNFα, IL-1, and IFNγ levels, and synovitis.[1]

Intracellular signaling and transcription factors

TNFα and IL-1 activate numerous intracellular signaling cascades, resulting in the transcription of genes coding for various cytokines and inflammatory mediators. The principal pathways involved are the p38 mitogen-activated protein kinase (p38 MAPK) and the c-Jun N-terminal kinase pathways. Several orally bioavailable small-molecule inhibitors of p38 MAPK are in clinical trials in RA.[1,10]

NF-κB family transcription factors are also highly involved in inflammatory responses. The efficacy of corticosteroids in controlling inflammation is largely based on inhibition of NF-κB transcriptional activity.[10] In addition, some of the beneficial effects of leflunomide and ciclosporin in RA are mediated via NF-κB inhibition. Small-molecule inhibitors of NF-κB are the focus of numerous preclinical and clinical research endeavors.[1]

Cytokines also promote transcription of proinflammatory genes by signaling through the JAK-STAT pathway.[11] After binding to cognate receptors, cytokines activate a family of cytoplasmic kinases called Janus activated kinases (JAKs). Activated JAKs then phosphorylate specific members of the family of signal transducers and activators of transcription (STAT). Orally active JAK inhibitors are now being studied in several clinical settings.[10]

> *Highlights in* **cytokine blockade** *2003–04*
>
> **WHAT'S IN?**
> - Etanercept
> - Infliximab
> - Adalimumab
> - Anakinra
> - Combination of methotrexate and anti-tumor necrosis factor (TNF)α agents
>
> **WHAT'S OUT?**
> - Combination of anti-TNFα and anti-interleukin (IL)-1 agents
> - Interferon β
> - IL-10
> - IL-4
> - IL-11

Unsuccessful cytokine targets

IL-4, IL-10 and IL-11 are cytokines that have exhibited promising anti-inflammatory activity in preclinical animal models. Unfortunately, several studies evaluating recombinant human IL-10 and IL-4 in RA failed to show significant clinical efficacy.[12] IL-11 has been shown to reduce the production of proinflammatory cytokines. However, a Phase II study of recombinant human IL-11 in RA showed only marginal benefits.

IFNβ downregulates TNFα and IL-1 production, and recombinant IFNβ has been approved to treat multiple sclerosis (USA and UK). In RA patients, therapy with recombinant IFNβ has not demonstrated significant efficacy.[13]

In several animal models of RA, improvement in the inflammation and bone destruction was noted when a combination of TNFα and

IL-1 inhibitors was administered.[14] In a placebo-controlled trial in RA patients who were also receiving methotrexate, the combination of etanercept and anakinra provided no treatment benefit over etanercept monotherapy.[15] In addition, the combination of cytokine inhibitors resulted in a higher incidence of serious infections. Thus, the combination of anti-TNFα and anti-IL-1 agents is not recommended for RA patients.

References

1. Smolen JS, Steiner G. Therapeutic strategies for rheumatoid arthritis. *Nat Rev Drug Discov* 2003; 2:473–88.

2. Shanahan JC, Moreland LW, Carter RH. Upcoming biologic agents for the treatment of rheumatic diseases. *Curr Opin Rheumatol* 2003;15:226–36.

3. Economides A, Carpenter L, Rudge J et al. Cytokine traps: multi-component, high-affinity blockers of cytokine action. *Nat Med* 2003;9: 47–52.

4. Choy EH, Hazelman B, Smith M et al. Efficacy of a novel PEGylated humanized anti-TNF fragment (CDP870) in patients with rheumatoid arthritis: a phase II double-blinded, randomized, dose-escalating trial. *Rheumatology (Oxford)* 2002;41:1133–7.

5. Doggrell SA. TACE inhibition: a new approach to treating inflammation. *Expert Opin Invest Drugs* 2002;11:1003–6.

6. Lovinger SP. Use of biologics for rheumatoid arthritis tempered by concerns over safety, cost. *JAMA* 2003;289:3229–30.

7. Kwon HJ, Cote TR, Cuffe MS et al. Case reports of heart failure after therapy with a tumor necrosis factor antagonist. *Ann Intern Med* 2003;138:807–11.

8. Choy EH, Isenberg DA, Carrod T et al. Therapeutic benefit of blocking interleukin-6 activity with an interleukin-6 receptor monoclonal antibody in rheumatoid arthritis: a randomized, double-blind, placebo-controlled, dose escalation trial. *Arthritis Rheum* 2002;46:3143–50.

9. Joosten L, Radstake T, Lubberts E et al. Association of IL-18 expression with enhanced levels of both IL-1β and TNF-α in knee synovial tissue of patients with rheumatoid arthritis. *Arthritis Rheum* 2003;48:339–47.

10. Tak PP, Firestein GS. NF-KappaB: a key role in inflammatory diseases. *J Clin Invest* 2001;107:7–11.

11. Changelian PS, Flanagan ME, Ball DJ et al. Prevention of oral allograft rejection by a specific Janus kinase 3 inhibitor. *Science* 2003; 302:875–8.

12. Keystone EC. Abandoned therapies and unpublished trials in rheumatoid arthritis. *Curr Opin Rheumatol* 2003;15:253–8.

13. Smeets TJM, Dayer JM, Kraan MC et al. The effects of interferon-β treatment on synovial inflammation and expression of metalloproteinases in patients with rheumatoid arthritis. *Arthritis Rheum* 2003;43:270–4.

14. Bendele AM, Chlipala ES, Scherrer J et al. Combination benefit of treatment with cytokine inhibitors interleukin-1 receptor antagonist and PEGylated soluble tumor necrosis factor receptor type I in animal models of rheumatoid arthritis. *Arthritis Rheum* 2000;43:2648–59.

15. Genovese MC, Cohen S, Moreland L et al. Combination therapy with etanercept and anakinra in the treatment of patients with rheumatoid arthritis failing methotrexate. *Arthritis Rheum*, in press.

Targeting lymphocytes using biological therapies

John D Isaacs PhD FRCP
School of Clinical Medical Sciences, University of Newcastle upon Tyne, UK

Cytokine blockade has provided a major therapeutic advance in the treatment of rheumatoid arthritis (RA) (see Townsend and Moreland, page 81). Ultimately, however, cytokine blockers require long-term administration, which is expensive and may be associated with tachyphylaxis and adverse effects related to chronic immunosuppression. In contrast, the optimal therapy would be one that could be administered for a brief period while providing long-term benefits. The capacity of lymphocyte-targeted therapies to 'switch off' disease in animal models of autoimmunity has been recognized for almost two decades.[1] Such approaches originally comprised the short-term administration of monoclonal antibodies (mAbs) against T-cell antigens such as CD4 and CD8, but subsequently extended to major histocompatibility complex (MHC)-blocking peptides, costimulation blockers and oral tolerance, to name just a few. The extension of these findings to the clinic could provide 'cures' for autoimmune diseases but, until recently, progress has been slow and erratic. For example, impressive results from small-scale open studies were difficult to replicate in the setting of the conventional clinical trial. Major hurdles included poor comprehension of the mechanism of action of such 'tolerogenic' therapies and an equally poor understanding of the tolerance mechanisms themselves.

Dominant tolerance

Interest in the clinical application of tolerogenic therapies has re-emerged and flourished over the past 5 years, largely as a consequence of the recognition of dominant tolerance mechanisms.[2] These involve so-called regulatory T cells, which actively and specifically suppress immune responses. It appears that various subsets of T cells actively patrol our immune systems and control unwanted autoreactivity. Although there has, so far, been no direct link to autoimmune disease in man, these are potentially very powerful cells. In the animal models referred to above, tolerogenic therapies are often associated with the emergence of regulatory T cells, which then contribute to long-term control of unwanted and pathological immune responses.

Costimulation blockade

A T cell requires at least two signals from an antigen-presenting cell to 'fire' and become activated. The first is received through the antigen-specific T-cell receptor and the second through costimulatory molecules, the most important of which is CD28. If the second signal is prevented, the T cell becomes tolerized and anergic. This is a powerful method for inducing tolerance in animal models and has recently been applied in the clinical setting.

CTLA4-Ig is a fusion protein comprising the extracellular domain of the T-cell surface protein CTLA4, fused to part of the constant region of human IgG_1. CTLA4 binds the same ligands as CD28, but with a higher affinity. Consequently, CTLA4-Ig competes with CD28 and prevents T cells from receiving 'second signals'. In a placebo-controlled, dose-finding study, RA patients receiving CTLA4-Ig alone had dose-dependent American College of Rheumatology (ACR) 20, 50 and 70 responses.[3] In a subsequent Phase IIB study, monthly CTLA4-Ig (2 mg or 10 mg) was given in combination with weekly low-dose methotrexate.[4] At 6 months, the ACR50 and 70 response rates were significantly higher in both active treatment groups compared with those in a placebo group. The group receiving 10 mg also showed a statistically superior ACR20 response rate, and overall responses in this group were comparable with those determined historically in patients receiving infliximab plus methotrexate. At 12 months, patients in this group continued to show benefit, as evidenced by improvements in physical function, and in quality of life.[5,6] Efficacy was also demonstrated when CTLA4-Ig was combined with etanercept in patients with an inadequate response to etanercept alone.[7,8]

While 6–12 months of therapy with CTLA4-Ig does not 'switch off' RA (as might be anticipated for a tolerogenic therapy), these studies clearly demonstrate the benefit of costimulation blockade. Another important costimulatory interaction is that between CD40L and CD40. The former is present on T cells and platelets, the latter on a variety of cell types, including antigen-presenting cells and B cells. There is considerable evidence that this molecular interaction is important for the production of pathogenic autoantibodies, as well as for T-cell activation. Anti-CD40L mAb has not yet been tested in RA. An open-label study in systemic lupus erythematosus, however, showed preliminary evidence for efficacy (reduced anti-double-stranded-DNA antibodies and hematuria, increased C3 complement levels), but it was terminated prematurely secondary to thromboembolic events.[9] The therapeutic effect may relate to reduced T-cell and consequent B-cell activation, the circulation of recipients containing fewer B cells secreting IgG and IgG anti-DNA antibodies.[10] Other work, however, suggests that this therapy may not interfere with costimulation but merely kills activated T cells.[11]

Targeting B cells

B cells clearly play an important role in RA pathogenesis. B cells and plasma cells are present in the inflamed synovium, and circulating autoantibodies may predate clinical disease by many years.[12] Furthermore, rheumatoid factor is a marker for more severe RA. In the 1990s, a convincing case was made that B cells may be the critical cell population controlling RA.[13] The availability of an anti-CD20 mAb (rituximab), which was highly effective at killing B cells, provided an opportunity to test this hypothesis. In the first two reports of this therapy, patients treated with short courses of rituximab developed profound and lasting improvements of their RA.[14,15] Interpretation was complicated because therapy was based around regimens used for lymphoma treatment, and incorporated both cyclophosphamide and high-dose corticosteroids. Slightly less impressive overall responses were observed in five patients who received rituximab alone.[16]

A recent Phase II study in partial responders to methotrexate compared continued methotrexate alone with rituximab alone, 1 g i.v. on days 1 and 15, and with the combinations of rituximab plus methotrexate, and rituximab plus cyclophosphamide, two doses of 750 mg i.v. All groups received a 17-day course of corticosteroid at the start of therapy. At 48 weeks, patients receiving rituximab plus methotrexate appeared to fare best, though responses were evident in all groups receiving rituximab.[17] Treatment was associated with a good safety profile despite a profound peripheral blood B-cell lymphopenia.[18] Intriguingly, rituximab leads to a decline in autoantibody levels without a significant change in antimicrobial antibodies.[19] Subsequent relapse is associated with rises in autoantibody levels.[19] B-cell blockade is now being studied in a number of potentially serologically mediated autoimmune diseases (see also pages 27 and 48).[20]

Other therapies in development

Anti-CD3 mAbs have been used therapeutically for many years, mainly for acute transplant rejection. The advent of safer anti-CD3 mAbs, however, has led to their evaluation in autoimmune disease. In a Phase I/II study, eight patients with psoriatic arthritis received 8–10 days of treatment with 4 mg huOKT3γ1(ala-ala), an Fc-modified anti-CD3 mAb. Six of seven patients who completed therapy demonstrated responses sustained beyond day 90.[21] When the same mAb was administered to people with recent-onset diabetes for 14 days, stabilization or improvement in pancreatic function was evident for more than 1 year in most recipients.[22] Recent evidence from animal models suggests that anti-CD3 therapy may lead to the generation of regulatory T cells in vivo,[23] which has generated considerable excitement.[24]

Effector T cells are presumed to coordinate tissue damage in autoimmunity and a therapy that preferentially targets this subset might provide a useful means to interrupt pathological immune responses. LFA3-Ig (alefacept) is a fusion protein between the first

> **Highlights in targeting lymphocytes using biological therapies 2003–04**
>
> **WHAT'S IN?**
> - Tolerance as a therapeutic goal
> - Costimulation blockade
> - Therapies that target B cells
> - The search for 'surrogate markers' of tolerance induction
>
> **WHAT'S OUT?**
> - The premise that autoimmunity can never be 'cured'

extracellular domain of LFA3 and part of human IgG_1. Because the ligand for LFA3 (CD2) is upregulated on effector and activated T cells, alefacept selectively kills these cells by antibody-dependent cell-mediated cytotoxicity.[25] In an exploratory study, 11 patients with psoriatic arthritis received alefacept, 7.5 mg/week, for 12 weeks.[26] At the end of the study, six patients had responded, which was mirrored by improvements in histological synovitis. Responders had higher baseline memory-effector (CD45RO+) T-cell counts in both peripheral blood and synovial tissue, and showed a significant reduction in response to therapy. Subsequently, 36 RA patients receiving methotrexate were randomized to alefacept, 3.75 mg/week or 7.5 mg/week for 12 weeks, or to placebo.[27] The groups receiving active treatment had superior ACR responses compared with the placebo group at both 14 and 24 weeks.

Surrogate markers
Both B and T cells provide promising targets for therapy of RA and other autoimmune diseases. Although we have not yet witnessed robust and long-lasting remissions in the absence of background

therapy, there is great anticipation in the field. One limitation to progress is our relatively poor understanding of tolerance induction and maintenance. This makes it impossible to monitor or guide therapy in terms of immunologic parameters that correlate with clinical improvement (equivalent to an 'immunological C-reactive protein'). A major research goal is the identification of such 'surrogate markers', which would revolutionize tolerogenic therapy.[28]

References

1. Waldmann H. Reprogramming the immune system. *Immunol Rev* 2002;185:227–35.

2. Graca L, Le Moine A, Cobbold SP et al. Dominant transplantation tolerance. Opinion. *Curr Opin Immunol* 2003;15:499–506.

3. Moreland LW, Alten R, Van den Bosch F et al. Costimulatory blockade in patients with rheumatoid arthritis: a pilot, dose-finding, double-blind, placebo-controlled clinical trial evaluating CTLA-4Ig and LEA29Y eighty-five days after the first infusion. *Arthritis Rheum* 2002;46:1470–9.

4. Kremer JM, Westhovens R, Leon M et al. Treatment of rheumatoid arthritis by selective inhibition of T cell activation with fusion protein CTLA4Ig. *N Engl J Med* 2003;349: 1907–15.

5. Tugwell P, Emery P, Kremer J et al. Physical function after treatment of CTLA4Ig (BMS-188667), a co-stimulation blocker, in patients with active rheumatoid arthritis using methotrexate. *Arthritis Rheum* 2003;48:S315.

6. Emery P, Russell A, Kremer J et al. Improvement in health-related quality of life with treatment of CTLA4Ig (BMS-188667), a selective co-stimulation modulator, over one year in patients with active rheumatoid arthritis using methotrexate. *Arthritis Rheum* 2003;48:S405.

7. Weinblatt M, Schiff M, Goldman M et al. A pilot, multi-center, randomized, double-blind, placebo controlled of a co-stimulation blocker CTLA4Ig (2mg/kg) given monthly in combination with etanercept in active rheumatoid arthritis. *Arthritis Rheum* 2002;46:S204.

8. Emery P, Williams GR, Li T et al. Improvement in health-related quality of life in patients with active rheumatoid arthritis: CTLA4Ig combined with etanercept plus placebo. *Arthritis Rheum* 2002;46:S514.

9. Boumpas DT, Furie R, Manzi S, on behalf of the BG9588 Lupus Nephritis Trial Group. A short course of BG9588 (anti-CD40 ligand antibody) improves serologic activity and decreases hematuria in patients with proliferative lupus glomerulonephritis. *Arthritis Rheum* 2003;48:719–27.

10. Huang W, Sinha J, Newman J et al. The effect of anti-CD40 ligand antibody on B cells in human systemic lupus erythematosus. *Arthritis Rheum* 2002;46:1554–62.

11. Monk NJ, Hargreaves RE, Marsh JE et al. Fc-dependent depletion of activated T cells occurs through CD40L-specific antibody rather than costimulation blockade. *Nat Med* 2003;9:1275–80.

12. Rantapää-Dahlqvist S, de Jong BAW, Berglin E et al. Antibodies against cyclic citrullinated peptide and IgA rheumatoid factor predict the development of rheumatoid arthritis. *Arthritis Rheum* 2003;48:2741–9.

13. Edwards JCW, Cambridge G, Abrahams VM. Do self-perpetuating B-lymphocytes drive human autoimmune disease? *Immunology* 1999;97:188–96.

14. Edwards JC, Cambridge G. Sustained improvement in rheumatoid arthritis following a protocol designed to deplete B lymphocytes. *Rheumatology (Oxford)* 2001;40:205–11.

15. Leandro MJ, Edwards JC, Cambridge G. Clinical outcome in 22 patients with rheumatoid arthritis treated with B lymphocyte depletion. *Ann Rheum Dis* 2002;61:883–8.

16. De Vita S, Zaja F, Sacco S et al. Efficacy of selective B cell blockade in the treatment of rheumatoid arthritis: Evidence for a pathogenetic role of B cells. *Arthritis Rheum* 2002;46:2029–33.

17. Emery P, Szczepanski L, Szechinski J et al. Sustained efficacy at 48 weeks after single treatment course of rituximab in patients with rheumatoid arthritis. *Arthritis Rheum* 2003;48:S439.

18. Szczepanski L, Szechinski J, Filipowicz-Sosnowska A. Safety data from 48 weeks follow-up of a randomized controlled trial of rituximab in patients with rheumatoid arthritis. *Arthritis Rheum* 2003;48:S121.

19. Cambridge G, Leandro MJ, Edwards JCW et al. Serologic changes following B lymphocyte depletion therapy for rheumatoid arthritis. *Arthritis Rheum* 2003;48:2146–54.

20. Silverman GJ, Weisman S. Rituximab therapy and autoimmune disorders: prospects for anti-B cell therapy. *Arthritis Rheum* 2003;48:1484–92.

21. Utset TO, Auger JA, Peace D et al. Modified anti-CD3 therapy in psoriatic arthritis: a phase I/II clinical trial. *J Rheumatol* 2002;29: 1907–13.

22. Herold KC, Hagopian W, Auger JA et al. Anti-CD3 monoclonal antibody in new-onset type 1 diabetes mellitus. *N Engl J Med* 2002;346: 1692–8.

23. Belghith M, Bluestone JA, Barriot S et al. TGF-beta-dependent mechanisms mediate restoration of self-tolerance induced by antibodies to CD3 in overt autoimmune diabetes. *Nat Med* 2003;9:1202–8.

24. Chatenoud L. CD3-specific antibody-induced active tolerance: From bench to bedside. *Nat Rev Immunol* 2003;3:123–32.

25. Cooper JC, Morgan G, Harding S et al. Alefacept selectively promotes NK cell-mediated deletion of CD45R0+ human T cells. *Eur J Immunol* 2003;33:666–75.

26. Kraan MC, van Kuijk AWR, Dinant HJ et al. Alefacept treatment in psoriatic arthritis: reduction of the effector T cell population in peripheral blood and synovial tissue is associated with improvement of clinical signs of arthritis. *Arthritis Rheum* 2002;46:2776–84.

27. Schneider M, Stahl H-D, Scaramucci J et al. Alefacept in subjects with active rheumatoid arthritis. *Arthritis Rheum* 2003;48:S654.

28. Isaacs JD, Waldmann H. Regaining self-control: regulation and immunotherapy. *Br J Rheumatol* 1998;37:926–9.

From genetics to functional genomics

Anna Lucia Bernardini MD **and Salvatore Albani** MD PhD
Departments of Pediatrics and Medicine, and the IACOPO Institute for Translational Medicine, University of California, San Diego, USA

Rheumatic diseases have a multifactorial origin, with genetic factors accounting for a significant component. There is general agreement on a model in which the accumulation or epistatic effects of multiple genes may predispose to many of these diseases, including rheumatoid arthritis (RA). RA is one of the most studied diseases of this group and it is the main focus of this brief review.

Methodology

Advances in the human genome project and the powerful association between the approaches taken in genomics, proteomics and functional immunology have determined a radical shift in the sequence of investigations in this field. The traditional epidemiological study, in which the representation of a given gene or cluster of genes in a certain disease is assessed, is now often preceded by genome-wide screens at increasing levels of sensitivity. This type of analysis uses all the available genotypic information to calculate the maximum logarithm of odds score (MLS) value at each point in the genome, and thereby generates MLS profiles along each chromosome. A positive MLS value indicates potential linkage. The peaks in these profiles, which may be referred to as 'hits', identify the most likely locations of disease-susceptibility genes.[1] Hits are then validated using additional techniques such as DNA sequencing, gene-expression profiling and functional studies. For example, microarray analysis (and other genomic or proteomic techniques) provides information on the expression of genes within target tissues that can then be 'mapped' to potential susceptibility loci identified by linkage studies.[2]

An autoimmune genotype?
Genome-wide screens have shown that autoimmunity is generally more prevalent among first- and second-degree relatives of patients with an index autoimmune disease.[3,4] Chromosomal regions linked to RA, for example, have previously been implicated in systemic lupus erythematosus (SLE), inflammatory bowel disease, multiple sclerosis and ankylosing spondylitis.[5] These data underscore the possibility that clinically distinct diseases may share common pathogenetic pathways.

Genes implicated in RA
A systematic whole-genome screen of affected sibling pairs from 182 UK families identified significant linkage around the major histocompatibility complex (MHC; human leukocyte antigen [HLA]) region on chromosome 6.[6] Other sites of nominal linkage were identified on various other chromosomes (3p, 4q, 7p, 10q, 14q, 16p, 21q and Xq by single-point analysis, and 1q and 14q by multipoint analysis). None of these reached the genome-wide threshold for significant linkage, though six of the regions had also been identified in previous studies. Combined analysis of two US datasets showed evidence for linkage at 6p21.3 (the HLA complex), 1p13, 1q43, 6q21, 10q21, 12q12, 17p13 and 18q21.[5,7]

Single-nucleotide polymorphisms (SNPs) are common genetic variants within genes and are distributed throughout the genome. They therefore serve as useful markers for genetic studies. SNPs may or may not affect the level of expression or function of the corresponding protein. This is why genetic studies employing SNPs may also focus on determining expression levels and other functional consequences.

PADI4. In a recent case–control linkage disequilibrium study, an RA-susceptibility haplotype was identified in *PADI4*, the gene encoding peptidylarginine deiminase type 4, which is one of the enzymes that change arginine into citrulline in proteins.[8,9] Citrullinated peptides have been implicated as autoantigens in RA, and *PADI4* has been shown to be expressed in the blood and synovial tissues of patients with RA.[9] The haplotype associated with RA affected the stability of *PADI4* transcripts. This haplotype was also associated with the presence of serum antibody against citrullinated peptide in people with RA. These findings provide a potentially important clue to the pathogenesis of RA.

HLA. Gene-expression patterns obtained by high-density microarrays, custom arrays, in-situ hybridization, and real-time PCR have been used to analyze HLA and other genetic contributions to RA.[10] This combination of powerful and innovative techniques has reinforced the notion that, among the immune response genes, HLA is strongly associated with susceptibility to, and the development and progression of many autoimmune diseases. The *HLA-DRB1*0401/0404* genotype is particularly associated with severe, erosive and seropositive RA,[11] though the precise role of HLA remains enigmatic. A recent, functional study suggested that promoter polymorphisms driving high expression of the relatively non-polymorphic *HLA-DRB4* alleles segregated with radiological damage in RA, whereas low *DRB4* expression was protective.[12] These effects appeared to be independent of *DRB1*04* alleles. RA patients also have an increased risk of cardiovascular disease that is independent of traditional cardiovascular risk factors. A recent study suggested that *HLA-DRB1* status was a predictor of impaired endothelial function in RA patients.[13] Overall, recent studies suggest that HLA is not particularly associated with the incidence of RA, but more with the progression and severity of the disease process.

Non-HLA genes. The function of non-HLA genes associated with autoimmunity may also prove difficult to resolve. A good example is the identification of the *IBD1* gene on chromosome 16 as *NOD2*. The study that showed the association of this gene with Crohn's disease was a landmark.[14] The disease-associated mutation reduces cellular activation in response to bacterial lipopolysaccharide. While at first sight this seems counterintuitive, it appears that other pathways may consequently be upregulated in diseased tissue, resulting in uncontrolled inflammation. Although many issues with respect to gene function and expression remain to be resolved, there is great optimism that important clinical applications will result directly from this work.[15,16]

Genetics and immunoregulation

Interleukin (IL)-10. Despite the changes to methodology outlined previously, the association study remains a widely used genetic approach. The frequency of specific polymorphisms located within or near candidate genes (inferred from the etiopathogenetic data available) is compared in disease and control populations. In this context, much interest has been focused on the tolerogenic cytokine IL-10. The gene encoding IL-10 is highly polymorphic with a number of SNPs in the promoter region and two microsatellite loci, *IL10.R* and *IL10.G*, 4 kb and 1.1 kb 5', respectively, from the transcription initiation site. Allele 2 of the *IL10.R* microsatellite (*IL10.R2*) is associated with increased IL-10 secretion, while *IL10.R3* is associated with reduced secretion. Associations between this locus and RA, juvenile idiopathic arthritis and SLE have been reported, but a recent study failed to confirm an association with RA in two ethnically diverse groups.[17]

Transforming growth factor (TGF)β1 is another immunoregulatory cytokine. A recent study employed both association and linkage analyses to determine whether genetic polymorphisms in or near the *TGFB1* locus were likely to play a role in susceptibility to or the severity of ankylosing spondylitis. Weak effects were demonstrated, but overall this study suggested that polymorphisms within the *TGFB1* gene played, at most, a small role in ankylosing spondylitis, and that other genes encoded on chromosome 19 were involved in susceptibility to the disease.[18]

Cytokine gene polymorphisms might be predicted to influence the clinical efficacy of cytokine blockade. A recent study correlated particular combinations of polymorphisms within the genes encoding tumor necrosis factor (TNF)α, IL-10, TGFβ and IL-1-receptor antagonist (IL-1Ra) with responsiveness to TNFα blockade. A particular combination of alleles influencing TNFα and IL-10 production was associated with a good response to etanercept, whereas a combination influencing TGFβ1 and IL-1Ra was associated with non-responsiveness.[19] It must, however, be emphasized that current knowledge does not yet justify large-scale genotyping for practical purposes. Further advances in technology and knowledge are needed to ensure the full transition from genetics into functional genomics.

CTLA4. Several studies have focused on polymorphisms within *CTLA4*, which encodes cytotoxic T lymphocyte antigen 4, a vital negative regulatory molecule of the immune system. In humans, a non-coding 6.1 kb 3' region of the *CTLA4* gene was shown to be associated with Graves' disease, autoimmune hypothyroidism and type 1 diabetes. The common allelic variant of this region was correlated with lower messenger RNA (mRNA) levels of the soluble alternative splice form of *CTLA4*, and similar findings were demonstrated in the NOD mouse diabetes model.[20] Quantitative alterations in *CTLA4* contribute to autoimmune tissue destruction.[20–22] *CTLA4* polymorphisms may also contribute to the pathogenesis of SLE and multiple sclerosis.[22,23]

These recent data provide critical information not only on the molecular basis of T cell inactivation by *CTLA4*, but also on the key requirements for the successful development of therapeutic strategies targeting this molecule.[24]

Indirect genetic effects in RA

DNA damage. Mutations in key genes controlling the cell cycle and/or function may also play a role in pathogenesis. Reactive oxygen species and reactive nitrogen species produced in the inflamed synovium have the potential to induce mutations in key genes, resulting in DNA damage. Normally this process is prevented by DNA mismatch repair (MMR), a system that maintains sequence fidelity during DNA replication and involves enzymes such as MutSalpha (hMSH2 and hMSH6) and MutSbeta (hMSH2 and hMSH3). When compared with osteoarthritic tissue, RA synovium

> **Highlights in genetics and genomics 2003–04**
>
> **WHAT'S IN?**
> - Genome-wide screens at high sensitivity
> - Multiplex family studies
> - Microsatellite analyses
> - Molecular biology and immunologic functional validation of hits
> - Translation of genetics into functional genomics
>
> **WHAT'S OUT?**
> - Reliance on epidemiological studies focused on genes chosen on presumptive assumptions as a first approach to genetic studies

showed extensive microsatellite instability (MSI), a sign of DNA damage, and low levels of hMSH6. Therefore, in RA synovium, oxidative stress not only creates free radicals that are potentially mutagenic, but also suppresses the mechanisms that limit the DNA damage.[25]

p53 **mutations.** A potential consequence of such DNA damage is the accumulation of somatic mutations in the *p53* gene. Clusters of *p53* mutant subclones, suggesting a clonal growth advantage, were identified in microdissected synovial tissue from RA patients. IL-6 gene expression is regulated by wild-type *p53*, and IL-6 mRNA expression was higher in regions of tissue with high rates of *p53* mutation. Thus, free radicals, via DNA damage, may endow RA synovial cells not only with a growth advantage, but also with a counterproductive increase in proinflammatory cytokine production.[26]

References

1. Altmuller J, Palmer LJ, Fischer G et al. Genomewide scans of complex human diseases: true linkage is hard to find. *Am J Hum Genet* 2001; 5:936–50.

2. Firneisz G, Zehavi I, Vermes C et al. Identification and quantification of disease-related gene clusters. *Bioinformatics* 2003;19:1781–6.

3. Prahalad S, Shear ES, Thompson SD et al. Increased prevalence of familial autoimmunity in simplex and multiplex families with juvenile rheumatoid arthritis. *Arthritis Rheum* 2002;46:1851–6.

4. Saila H, Savolainen A, Kauppi M et al. Occurrence of chronic inflammatory rheumatic diseases among parents of multiple offspring affected by juvenile idiopathic arthritis. *Clin Exp Rheumatol* 2003;21:263–5.

5. Jawaheer D, Seldin MF, Amos CI et al. A genomewide screen in multiplex rheumatoid arthritis families suggests genetic overlap with other autoimmune diseases. *Am J Hum Genet* 2001;68:927–36.

6. MacKay K, Eyre S, Myerscough A et al. Whole-genome linkage analysis of rheumatoid arthritis susceptibility loci in 252 affected sibling pairs in the United Kingdom. *Arthritis Rheum* 2002;46:582–4.

7. Jawaheer D, Seldin MF, Amos CI et al. Screening the genome for rheumatoid arthritis susceptibility genes: a replication study and combined analysis of 512 multicase families. *Arthritis Rheum* 2003;48:906–16.

8. Suzuki A, Yamada R, Chang X et al. Functional haplotypes of *PADI4*, encoding citrullinating enzyme peptidylarginine deiminase 4, are associated with rheumatoid arthritis. *Nat Genet* 2003;4:395–402.

9. Yamada R, Suzuki A, Chang X et al. Peptidylarginine deiminase type 4: identification of a rheumatoid arthritis-susceptible gene. *Trends Mol Med* 2003;9:503–8.

10. Barton A, Ollier W. Genetic approaches to investigation of rheumatoid arthritis. *Curr Opin Rheumatol* 2002;14:260–9.

11. Wagner U, Kaltenhauser S, Pierer M et al. Prospective analysis of the impact of HLA-DR and -DQ on joint destruction in recent-onset rheumatoid arthritis. *Rheumatology (Oxford)* 2003;42:553–62.

12. Heldt C, Listing J, Sozeri O et al. Differential expression of HLA class 2 genes associated with disease susceptibility and progression in rheumatoid arthritis. *Arthritis Rheum* 2003; 48:2779–87.

13. Gonzalez-Juanatey C, Testa A, Garcia-Castelo A et al. HLA-DRB1 status affects endothelial function in treated patients with rheumatoid arthritis. *Am J Med* 2003;114: 647–52.

14. Ogura Y, Bonen DK, Inohara N et al. A frameshift mutation in *NOD2* associated with susceptibility to Crohn's disease. *Nature* 2001; 411:603–6.

15. Satsangi J, Morecroft J, Shah NB, Nimmo E. Genetics of inflammatory bowel disease: scientific and clinical implications. *Best Prac Res Clin Gastroenterol* 2003;17:3–18.

16. Girardin SE, Hugot JP, Sansonetti PJ. Lessons from Nod2 studies: towards a link between Crohn's disease and bacterial sensing. *Trends Immunol* 2003;24:652–8.

17. MacKay K, Milicic A, Lee D et al. Rheumatoid arthritis susceptibility and interleukin 10: a study of two ethnically diverse populations. *Rheumatology (Oxford)* 2003; 42:149–53.

18. Jaakkola E, Crane AM, Laiho K et al. The effect of transforming growth factor β1 gene polymorphisms in ankylosing spondylitis. *Rheumatology (Oxford)* 2004; 43:32–8.

19. Padyukov J, Lampa M, Heimburger S et al. Genetic markers for the efficacy of tumour necrosis factor blocking therapy in rheumatoid arthritis. *Ann Rheum Dis* 2003;62:526–9.

20. Ueda H, Howson JM, Esposito L et al. Association of the T-cell regulatory gene *CTLA4* with susceptibility to autoimmune disease. *Nature* 2003;423:506–11.

21. Maszyna F, Hoff H, Kunkel D et al. Diversity of clonal T cell proliferation is mediated by differential expression of CD152 (*CTLA-4*) on the cell surface of activated individual T lymphocytes. *J Immunol* 2003;171:3459–66.

22. Alizadeh M, Babron MC, Birebent B et al. Genetic interaction of CTLA-4 with HLA-DR15 in multiple sclerosis patients. *Ann Neurol* 2003;54:119–22.

23. Liu MF, Wang CR, Chen PC, Fung LL. Increased expression of soluble cytotoxic T-lymphocyte-associated antigen-4 molecule in patients with systemic lupus erythematosus. *Scand J Immunol* 2003;57:568–72.

24. Baroja ML, Madrenas J. Viewpoint: therapeutic implications of CTLA-4 compartmentalization. *Am J Transplant* 2003;3:919–26.

25. Lee SH, Chang DK, Goel A et al. Microsatellite instability and suppressed DNA repair enzyme expression in rheumatoid arthritis. *J Immunol* 2003;170:2214–20.

26. Yamanashi Y, Boyle DL, Rosengren S et al. Regional analysis of p53 mutations in rheumatoid arthritis synovium. *Proc Natl Acad Sci USA* 2002;99:10025–30.

Mesenchymal progenitor cells

Elena Jones PhD, **Anne English** FIBMS and **Dennis McGonagle** PhD FRCPI
Rheumatology Research Unit, University of Leeds, UK

Mesenchymal progenitor cells (MPCs) are highly proliferative clonogenic cells that can produce bone, cartilage, fat and muscle. The presence of MPCs in adult tissue was discovered over four decades ago by Friedenstein and colleagues;[1] they demonstrated that particular bone-marrow cells that were adherent and had a morphology of fibroblasts could form histologically normal bone and cartilage following transplantation in mice. From a historical perspective, the subsequent research into MPC biology was, for the most part, performed by hematologists, and to a lesser extent by specialists in bone biology and orthopedics.

For nearly two decades there has been much speculation and hypothesizing about the role of putative MPCs in rheumatology. Primitive-looking mesenchymal cells have been noted at sites of cartilage erosion in both experimental and human studies, and a role for these in the pathogenesis of rheumatoid arthritis (RA) has been suggested.[2] An unusual cell – termed a pannocyte – has been isolated from articular cartilage, and has been likened to a stem cell.[3] These observations have culminated in the idea that RA may be initiated and perpetuated by mesenchymal stem cells.[4] In the case of osteoarthritis (OA), new bone formation with osteophytosis and bone sclerosis is strong evidence for a role for MPCs, though direct proof is lacking.

Bone-marrow MPCs

Starting from the pioneering work of Friedenstein, bone-marrow MPCs have been known to adhere to plastic or glass and to be capable of proliferating and forming distinct colonies of fibroblasts in culture (hence their old name, fibroblast-colony-forming units or CFU-Fs). The next major breakthrough came with the discovery of the Stro-1 antigen as a unique marker of human bone marrow CFU-Fs and subsequent confirmation in vitro that all bone-marrow osteogenic progenitors are confined to this fraction.[5,6] Another major milestone was a publication by Pittenger et al., who devised and standardized in-vitro assays of trilineage differentiation and proved the multipotentiality of MPCs at the single-cell level.[7]

Our group has demonstrated that bone-marrow MPCs belong to a non-hematopoietic mesenchymal (CD45-low) fraction, and express a multitude of markers specific for fibroblasts (CD13, CD90, CD10, D7-FIB, CD105 and others).[8] They also have a characteristic expression of low-affinity nerve-growth-factor receptor (LNGFR), which has been described in fetal mesenchyme, that distinguishes them from common skin fibroblasts. Some of these findings have since been corroborated and extended by Simmons's group.[9]

Rheumatoid arthritis

Based on the observation that bone morphogenetic protein-1A (BMPR1A) is expressed in embryonic mesenchymal tissue,[10] it has been presumed that synovial-tissue expression of this marker indicated the presence of primitive MPCs. In humans, mesenchymal cells positive for BMPR1A have been reported to account for up to 25% of synovial lining cells.[11] A similar study in rats suggested that MPCs might be involved in the initiation of arthritis.[12] Based on some limited immunophenotypic studies of peripheral blood, it has also been suggested that mesenchymal cells might circulate in arthritis. However, these reports only provided some immunophenotypic data – they did not show the cells to be multipotential and clonogenic, as is required to fulfill the current MPC definition.

Luyten's group has shown that normal synovial tissue contains highly proliferative and multipotential MPCs.[13] One of the conclusions was that the in-vivo topography and number of MPCs in the synovial tissue needs to be defined. Although it is thought that in-vivo proliferation of synovial lining cells contributes to synovial hyperplasia,[14] it is possible that ingression of MPCs that have undergone cell division elsewhere contributes to the hyperplasia.

RA is a polyarticular disease – an attractive hypothesis is that MPCs circulating from the bone marrow can colonize multiple joints, accounting for the widespread distribution of disease. However, several studies aiming to identify and enumerate circulating MPCs in peripheral and cord blood produced inconsistent data.[15–18] MPCs may truly be absent from blood or occur at a very low frequency. Or there may be fundamental differences in the biology of circulating cells (such as inability to adhere), that have meant that they have not been detected in the majority of studies. To date, there are insufficient data to support the assertion that MPCs have a major role in the pathogenesis of RA.

Osteoarthritis

One would expect to find MPCs in OA because attempted joint regeneration and repair is a prominent feature of the disease. Conversely, cartilage defects never undergo spontaneous repair, suggesting a parallel defect of MPCs in OA. We have evaluated the synovial fluid in both OA and RA for the presence of MPCs, to evaluate whether synovial fluid MPCs play a role in lining-layer hyperplasia (RA), and/or attempted microdamage repair of the superficial layers of articular cartilage (OA).[19] We noted that a population of cells phenotypically and morphologically identical to bone-marrow MPCs occurred in arthritic synovial fluid. These cells were rare in both early and late RA, giving little evidence to support a role in the pathogenesis. However, they were significantly more numerous in OA, indicating either shedding from diseased joint structures or, possibly, some role in attempted joint repair. In another study investigating MPCs in OA, Murphy et al. showed that similar cells from the bone marrow of patients could make good-quality bone in vitro, but could not form cartilage.[20]

Articular cartilage has been explored for the presence of MPC activity, and two independent groups have demonstrated that human chondrocytes, dedifferentiated in culture, acquire a trilineage plasticity.[21,22] Moreover, Dell'Accio et al. showed that proliferation in culture (and associated dedifferentiation) was not required for myogenic differentiation of cartilage-derived cells.[23] Although evidence exists for a multipotent progenitor population in the superficial layer of cartilage,[24] it has not yet been proven at the single-cell level and it remains uncertain whether cartilage contains a subpopulation of MPCs phenotypically distinct from chondrocytes. At this stage, a direct reprogramming of a chondrocyte into a more primitive MPC, occurring under conditions of stress or injury, cannot be ruled out.

Other joint structures containing MPCs

Periostium also contains chondroprogenitors.[25] It is possible that such cells may have a role in perostitis and periarticular osteophytosis. The recent demonstration of MPCs in fat tissue from sites of lipoaspiration was both a surprise and of great interest.[26] Investigators have since grown MPC cultures from the infrapatellar fat pad.[27] The role of such cells and their ability to migrate to other joint sites remain to be established. A recent paper has shown that tendon contains MPCs, indicating that such cells could have an important role in homeostasis and repair.[28]

Every joint structure so far evaluated has been found to contain MPC activity, albeit activity not yet pinned to a specific cell subpopulation. The challenge now is to prove whether or not a 'mature' cell within these structures could reprogram to become an MPC (i.e. acquire primitive properties) under certain microenvironmental stimuli.

MPCs in therapy

There is increasing interest in the role of MPCs in regenerative medicine and there have been a number of attempts to use MPCs to repair damaged bone and cartilage.[29–31] When culture-expanded MPCs were used to repair articular cartilage defects, the results were disappointing.[30,31] There was poor integration of MPC-loaded constructs into defects and the tissue formed was invariably

> ### *Highlights in* **mesenchymal progenitor cells** *2003–04*
>
> #### WHAT'S IN?
> - Demonstration of mesenchymal progenitor cell (MPC) activity in several connective tissues within joint, suggestive of potential innate regenerative capacity
> - Investigation of the in-vivo biology of tissue-resident MPCs at the level of single cells
> - Standardization of assays for MPC evaluation from different sites
>
> #### WHAT'S OUT?
> - The field is too new to exclude existing dogma or theories

fibrocartilagenous or scar tissue.[30] The rational use of MPCs in joint repair requires greater knowledge of normal MPC physiology. In addition, the quality of the cell-supporting scaffold is a critical issue. It should be biodegradable and should not interfere with appropriate lineage differentiation within a construct at the site of bone, cartilage or ligament defect. Further, the optimal cocktail of growth factors required for appropriate lineage commitment (and its optimal delivery) needs to be ascertained. The eventual use of MPCs, tissue scaffolds and growth factors in cell therapy may remain problematic because of the many distinct commercial interests vested in the molecules and techniques.

Some groups are injecting MPCs into the circulation in the hope that they will home to sites of disease and mediate tissue repair. This strategy has recently been used for experimentally induced myocardial infarction; systemically administered MPCs were incorporated into the marginal tissue of infarcts, though more impressive MPC integration followed direct intraventricular administration.[32] The effects may have been caused by homing of circulating donor MPCs or they may reflect a 'reprogramming' of resident muscle cells at the site of the damage.[33] Although systemic delivery of MPCs raises the possibility of their use in gene therapy for the rheumatic diseases, many important questions of basic

References

1. Friedenstein AJ, Chalakhyan RK, Latsinik NV et al. Stromal cells responsible for transferring the microenvironment of the hemopoietic tissues. *Transplantation* 1974; 17:331–40.

2. Jorgensen C, Noel D, Gross G. Could inflammatory arthritis be triggered by progenitor cells in the joints? *Ann Rheum Dis* 2002;61:6–9.

3. Zvaifler NJ, Tsai V, Alsalameh S et al. Pannocytes: distinctive cells found in rheumatoid arthritis articular cartilage erosions. *Am J Pathol* 1997;150:1125–38.

4. Corr M, Zvaifler NJ. Mesenchymal precursor cells. *Ann Rheum Dis* 2002;61:3–5.

5. Simmons P, Torok-Storb B. Identification of stromal cell precursors in human bone marrow by a novel monoclonal antibody, Stro-1. *Blood* 1991;78:55–62.

6. Gronthos S, Graves SE, Ohta S et al. The Stro-1+ fraction of adult human bone marrow contains the osteogenic precursors. *Blood* 1994;84:4164–73.

7. Zannettino AC, Harrison K, Joyner CJ et al. Molecular cloning of the cell surface antigen identified by the osteoprogenitor-specific monoclonal antibody, HOP-26. *J Cell Biochem* 2003;89:56–66.

8. Jones EA, Kinsey SE, English A et al. Isolation and characterization of bone marrow multipotential mesenchymal progenitor cells. *Arthritis Rheum* 2002;46:3349–60.

9. Gronthos S, Zannettino ACW, Hay SJ et al. Molecular and cellular characterisation of highly purified stromal stem cells derived from human bone marrow. *J Cell Sci* 2003;116:1827–35.

10. Rosen V. Signalling pathways in skeletal formation. A role for BMP receptors. In: Crombrugge B, ed. *Molecular and Developmental Biology of Cartilage*. Ann NY Acad Sci No 785, 1996:56–9.

11. Marinova-Mutavshieva L, Taylor P, Funa K et al. Mesenchymal cells expressing bone morphogenic protein receptors are present in the rheumatoid arthritis joint. *Arthritis Rheum* 2000;43:2046–55.

12. Marinova-Mutafchieva L, Williams RO, Funa K et al. Inflammation is preceded by tumor necrosis factor-dependent infiltration of mesenchymal cells in experimental arthritis. *Arthritis Rheum* 2002;46:507–13.

13. De Bari C, Dell'Accio F, Tylzanowsky P et al. Multipotent mesenchymal stem cells from adult human synovial membrane. *Arthritis Rheum* 2001;44:1928–42.

14. Qu Z, Garcia CH, O'Rourke LM et al. Local proliferation of fibroblast-like synoviocytes contributes to synovial hyperplasia. Results of proliferating cell nuclear antigen/cyclin, c-myc, and nucleolar organizer region. *Arthritis Rheum* 1994;37:212–20.

15. Kuznetsov SA, Mankani MH, Gronthos S et al. Circulating skeletal stem cells. *J Cell Biol* 2001;153:1133–9.

16. Zvaifler NJ, Marinova-Mutafchieva L, Adams G et al. Mesenchymal precursor cells in the blood of normal individuals. *Arthritis Res* 2000; 2:477–88.

17. Goodwin HS, Bicknese AR, Chien SN et al. Multilineage differentiation activity by cells isolated from umbilical cord blood: expression of bone, fat, and neural markers. *Biol Blood Marrow Transplant* 2001;7:581–8.

18. Wexler SA, Donaldson C, Denning-Kendall P et al. Adult bone marrow is a rich source of human mesenchymal 'stem' cells but umbilical cord and mobilized adult blood are not. *Br J Haematol* 2003;121:368–74.

19. Jones EA, English A, Henshaw K et al. Enumeration and phenotypic characterization of synovial fluid multipotential mesenchymal progenitor cells in inflammatory and degenerative arthritis. *Arthritis Rheum*;in press.

20. Murphy JM, Dixon K, Beck S et al. Reduced chondrogenic and adipogenic activity of mesenchymal stem cells from patients with advanced osteoarthritis. *Arthritis Rheum* 2002;46:704–14.

21. Tallheden T, Dennis JE, Lennon DP et al. Phenotypic plasticity of human articular chondrocytes. *J Bone Joint Surg Am* 2003;85(Suppl 2):93–100.

22. Barbero A, Ploegert S, Heberger M et al. Plasticity of clonal populations of dedifferentiated adult human articular chondrocytes. *Arthritis Rheum* 2003;48:1315–25.

23. Dell'Accio F, De Bari C, Luyten FP. Microenvironment and phenotypic stability specify tissue formation by human articular cartilage-derived cells in vivo. *Exp Cell Res* 2003;287:16–27.

24. Hayes AJ, MacPhearson S, Morrison H et al. The development of articular cartilage: evidence for an appositional growth mechanism. *Anat Embryol* 2001;203:469–79.

25. De Bari C, Dell'Accio F, Luyten FP. Human periosteum-derived cells maintain phenotypic stability and chondrogenic potential throughout expansion regardless of donor age. *Arthritis Rheum* 2001;44:85–95.

26. Zuk PA, Zhu M, Ashjian P et al. Human adipose tissue is a source of multipotent stem cells. *Mol Biol Cell* 2002;13:4279–95.

27. Wickham MQ, Erickson GR, Gimble JM et al. Multipotent stromal cells derived from the infrapatellar fat pad of the knee. *Clin Orthop* 2003;412:196–212.

28. Salingcarnboriboon R, Yoshitake H, Tsuji K et al. Establishment of tendon-derived cell lines exhibiting pluripotent mesenchymal stem cell-like property. *Exp Cell Res* 2003; 287:289–300.

29. Bruder SP, Fox BS. Tissue engineering of bone. Cell based strategies. *Clin Orthop* 1999;367(Suppl):S68–83.

30. Gelse K, von der Mark K, Aigner T et al. Articular cartilage repair by gene therapy using growth factor-producing mesenchymal cells. *Arthritis Rheum* 2003;48:430–41.

31. Hunziker EB. Articular cartilage repair: basic science and clinical progress. A review of the current status and prospects. *Osteoarthritis Cartilage* 2002;10:432–63

32. Barbash IM, Chouraqui P, Baron J et al. Systemic delivery of bone marrow-derived mesenchymal stem cells to the infarcted myocardium: feasibility, cell migration, and body distribution. *Circulation* 2003;108: 863–8.

33. Prockop DJ, Gregory CA, Spees JL. One strategy for cell and gene therapy: harnessing the power of adult stem cells to repair tissues. *Proc Natl Acad Sci USA* 2003;100 (Suppl 1):11917–23.